Fatigue

One Woman's Recipe for Living
with M.E./Chronic Fatigue
and Improving Quality of Life

Sarah Warde

I dedicate this book to my son Sam. Your unwavering support and encouragement is like gold dust. You are my sunshine xx.

CONTENTS

ACKNOWLEDGEMENTS

I am incredibly lucky and grateful to have had so many wonderful people in my life. First on the list is always my father, John Christopher Thompson. He was/is my mentor. He was the most loving and kind man. He passed when I was 19 but remains in my heart always. I turn to him regularly.

Next is my mother Marie Thompson (Heffernan) who I turn to for strength. She backs me from above.

In the here and now I have the most supportive and loving Husband Jim, and son Sam. I would be nowhere without them as they have been my strength. I am a very lucky woman.

Next are my brother and sisters and my friends. Thank you for being there for me always.

The most influential people in the management of this condition are: Dr. Pearce, whose quick decisive action saved me back in 2001; Dr. Andrew Kelly who has been an incredible support throughout, and Dr. Mary Ryan who has been my specialist for many years now. Her kindness and directness really helped me. Next is Declan Carroll from the Irish ME Trust. Thank you for all your support. Madge O' Callaghan who is a writer and has helped me enormously with the editing and tweaking of this book.

And to all the other people who have been there for me and helped me manage this wonderful thing called life.

Thank you, x

I CAN CREATE AN INTERNAL PLACE OF PEACE AND
SAFETY NO MATTER WHERE I AM. I JUST HAVE TO
BREATHE AND RELAX MY THOUGHTS.

FOREWORD

Travel and documentation of the journey through books or a diary is an exciting part of life and always a joy to do and read. My father, Dr Denis Dooley OBE, kept a diary when he walked to Versailles in France. Hilaire Belloc in The Path to Rome writes about his physical as well as his spiritual journey.

Life is a journey and documentation of your path is often full of wisdom. Sarah has produced a very informative, interesting as well as an enjoyable book on her journey and needs to be congratulated for her dedication to helping others – well done.

I have known Sarah for over 40 years as her brother-in-law and followed her journey with interest. As documented in her book there have been ups and downs which Sarah has gone through so well and she has always learnt and gained from the experience and this is so inspiring to read about.

About 17 million individuals worldwide suffer from the debilitating condition of M.E./CFS – this is a huge number and probably an underestimate. Symptoms are varied and there are no specific diagnostic tests. Treatment depends on your individual symptoms. Self-help is often a central element

Travelling alone can be lonely, difficult, and stressful. To have a companion on your journey is often so helpful and not only can ease the pain but also you can learn from the experience of others – Sarah is your travel companion on this journey. This book will help so many. It should be essential reading for all sufferers who will learn from her excellent tips and advice. It should also be on the bookshelf and read by all health professionals involved in care – understanding the paths others have travelled can be so informative.

Congratulations Sarah for sharing your journey, experience, and self-help tips in such a clear and informative way - you will help many

Dr Michael Dooley MMS FFSRH FRCOG: Consultant Gynaecologist Dorset UK and Fellow of the Royal College of Obstetricians and Gynaecologists.

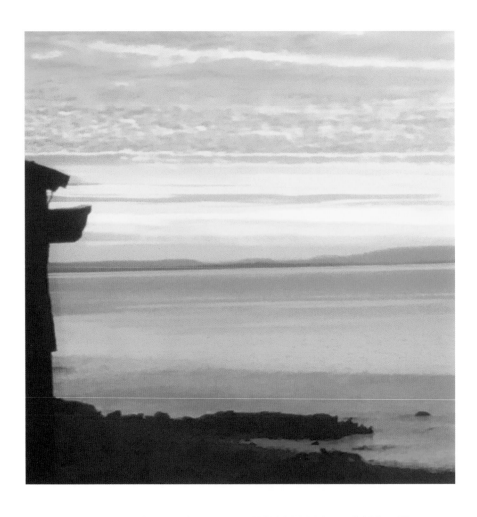

I CAN BE CHANGED BY WHAT HAPPENS TO ME
BUT I REFUSE TO BE REDUCED BY IT.

HOW IT ALL BEGAN

This new chapter of my life started in 2001. Before that things were a lot different. I was married with a young son, worked full time and life was good. I was a fun-loving young woman who enjoyed getting out. I had always been a highly active person whose nick name was Smiley. I was called Speedy when skiing on the slopes. When out with my friends I loved to dance until the last song. The word lazy was definitely not in my vocabulary.

Then it all changed. I can remember where I was and what I was doing. That morning was like any other. I got up and Sam and I had breakfast, my husband had already left for work earlier. I dropped my son to the Creche and headed to work. I had my gear bag in the back of the car so had planned to head for a swim as usual that evening. I was very fit and swam a couple of times a week. While at work I got a cough that felt very unusual and sore in my chest.

Now I'm not one to go to the doctor regularly but there was something hugely different about this so I said I would get it checked out. Later that day I left the doctor's office with antibiotics, steroids, and inhalers, which I thought, at the time was a bit over the top. I was told to remain home for two weeks. I did what I was told and didn't feel any better. In fact, I felt a lot worse, but thought "sure I've done what I was told I will be fine".

I am only telling this story so that anyone reading this can learn from my mistakes.

I had developed an annoying cough, a continuous tickle in my throat which I paid no attention to. I believed it would just go away eventually. I was taking lots of medicines, wasn't I?

When I went back to work, things took a turn for the worse. The cough got worse because I was moving around more. My colleagues started to look at me. I reassured them I was taking my medications and that it was probably the tail end of my sickness. At this stage I had developed an annoying pain in my side which I thought was a pulled muscle.

I needed to go downstairs to the Engineering section to give them drawings and on the way up the stairs the coughing escalated into coughing fits. My colleagues were concerned so I rang my GP. I told them something was very wrong, but they had no available appointments for me. Shortly after that I coughed so hard one of my ribs broke. I could not move. My friend brought me to the University Hospital Limerick, and I was admitted.

On day 2 of the Hospital stay I was in my room. It was late afternoon, and I started coughing but it didn't stop. I ended up leaning over the side of the bed on my tummy, violently coughing and gasping for air. At this stage, I was terrified, as the choking feeling left me in no doubt that something was definitely not right. A nurse passed the door and said, "I can hear you; I can hear you" and she kept going. I'd been coughing for so long that they were taking little notice. Once the episode passed my fear and anger took over. I pressed the call bell. Someone eventually came to my room. I was polite but firm and requested a second opinion as soon as possible. I knew I was in trouble.

The new doctor, a respiratory specialist arrived. He came in with his team and took one look at me and checked me out quickly, no more than a minute. Everything changed in that minute. Suddenly, everyone was being given swift, firm instructions from the doctor and all the team were running around in every direction. Some around me and others out the door to get what they needed. He informed them in no uncertain terms that not only had I one broken rib but two! The coughing was caused by asthma, which I never had before. I had Pneumonia in both my lungs. I was given lots of medications over the next 48 hours and soon after sent home to recuperate.

I was so ill at the time I didn't realise that this doctor saved my life. If I had not asked for a second opinion things would have gone very differently. He informed me that I was "a very lucky girl".

I was very fragile when I got home, and things were hugely different. My body was not responding well to the experience. The medication they gave me and the damage the incident had caused my body, started to unravel itself.

Talking for any length of time was proving difficult. I would tire very quickly. After 5 minutes my jaws would tire and ache, and my eyes would become very heavy. Holding a conversation was a nightmare. My concentration would drift, and my comprehension became muddled. Brain fog was a big issue. I would miss chunks of the conversation and my forehead and eyes would ache from the fatigue and feel very heavy.

Remember I was a fit young woman in her early 30s at this stage who used to swim 50 lengths of a pool with not even a panting breath. This "Mysterious Virus" as they called it, had knocked the stuffing out of me.

Migraines and nausea were a huge problem for the next fifteen years. The amount of times I was asked was I pregnant was funny. That would have really thrown the cat amongst the pigeons. The migraines and nausea surfaced after I came out of hospital back in 2001. If I did not stop when the warning signs of the fatigue started, they popped up keeping me in place. I needed to make several hospital visits to manage the pain. Before all this I'd talk for Ireland and never tire. I rarely suffered headaches let alone migraines.

I tried to push the boundaries a little further but each time I would end up back to square one, taking the Antibiotic my specialist instructed me to take to stop the chest infection travelling into my lungs. The antibiotics were strong, but they did the trick. I ended up taking them nearly every six weeks. Little by little things started to heal and I felt my body get stronger.

Four months later, I began to see light at the end of the tunnel. I started to push myself a little more and went to a party. This was at night and I stayed out till 1am. It was a great night out and my first late one since my hospital visit. I was telling friends I was feeling a lot better and would be returning to work shortly. I thought I was flying it. Unfortunately, my body had other plans. The high became a low very quickly and before I knew where I was, my chest had struck again. I was back on antibiotics which resulted in having absolutely no energy again. I was gutted.

My GP advised me to put off going back to work for another while. I was upset about that as I loved the social interaction. It took me three weeks to get to a stage where I could move through the house without my body feeling like lead. I started getting out for walks again. Starting with five minutes and building up to fifteen minutes maximum as instructed by my GP. Some days I could do it, others not at all. I had to listen to my body and heed what it was telling me.

I waited another few months before I attempted to bring up the subject of going back to work. At this stage it was the end of April 2002. I was sure this was the turning point and that my life would return to normal very soon.

I went to talk to my GP and let him know that I had lined up an interview for a nice easy job. Nothing too stressful or strenuous to start with. He agreed and asked me to do one test before signing me off. I was happy with this plan.

The following day I started the challenge. It was an exercise test. I had to go to the gym every second day for a week and get on the treadmill for twenty minutes. The first day went well. I left with a smile on my face. Two days later when I went back the tide had turned and my legs felt like lead. I could barely move, and I could not finish the twenty minutes. I was gutted. I never got back to the gym on the last day as I ended up back with the GP. My glands were swollen, and my throat was very sore. I was sent to a unit in the University Hospital Limerick. I knew what was happening and I knew the infection would travel fast into my lungs as it had before back in November. I asked the doctor to get in touch with the specialist that had treated me in November but was refused. I was given antibiotics and sent home. The following day I went back into the hospital. I felt much worse and I knew I was in trouble. They gave me a stronger antibiotic and sent me home again. I had requested them to contact my specialist but was refused again!

The day after that was no joke. I arrived at the hospital and went to the unit. I went through the doors and collapsed. It had taken all I had to get into the hospital. Before I knew what was happening, I was placed on a bed and hooked up to an IV. The doctor who refused to contact the specialist, that had treated me in November was very apologetic. What could I do but just lie there and look at him in disbelief and think "Why oh why, didn't you listen to me"? Hopefully, he learnt a lesson that patients need to be listened to. After lying there for a while my husband, Jim, arrived. He was not happy and expressed it.

After a few hours, the nurse told me that I was an invalid now and that I had been treated for a severe case of pneumonia. I had to go home and get complete rest for a few weeks and not to push myself at all or I would end up back in the hospital again. I did not want that.

I had been in this situation back in November, so I knew the drill. I soon discovered that the nurse was not exaggerating. Things were vastly different. My body had deteriorated a great deal since the last time in hospital. I was much more sluggish now. There was no spring in my step. The migraines were crippling. Sometimes they would last for days. They also brought nausea with them and that was rotten.

Not long after that, about six weeks, I was diagnosed with Myalgic Encephalomyelitis (M.E.), also known as Chronic Fatigue Syndrome (CFS), some like to call it Post Viral Fatigue.

M.E./CFS is a medical condition characterised, by long-term fatigue and other persistent symptoms that limit a person's ability to carry out ordinary daily activities.

Nobody understood what I was going through, I barely understood myself. It is difficult for family and friends to deal with the drastic changes. There was talk of depression which I knew in my gut wasn't the case but to put my mind and others at ease I went to see a top psychiatrist. I wanted to make sure I was not depressed. After talking to the psychiatrist, he agreed I was no more depressed than he was and that I had a condition nobody understood called M.E./CFS. He reassured me that it was real and recognised by the World Health Organisation (WHO) as a neurological condition, and to go and take it easy and heed to the advice my doctor was giving me. He acknowledged that I was a strong person and gave me a few pointers around the way

I was thinking and how to tweak things a little and before I left he told me "Don't let anyone diminish you".

I appreciated his understanding and went home content in knowing depression wasn't something I needed to worry about. I had a little secondary depression, which I kept an eye on but most of us get that. It is brought about by frustration and annoyance of the situation I was in. I took his advice and tweaked a few things in my thought process and that helped.

Time went by and I never got back to feeling I could go back to work. My GP, Dr. Andrew Kelly, was an amazing support. He agreed I was definitely not up to it.

My immune system was shot as I had been treated for pneumonia twice within six months, which had left my body rattled.

Now I am over nineteen years down the road and if I knew then what I know now, things could have been a lot better regarding dealing with this condition. That is the reason I am writing this book. I've made a lot of mistakes with overdoing it (not recommended at all!) and trying to get back to work and each time this condition, M.E./ CFS would put me in my place. If this book helps you change even one thing for the better, then I am delighted I wrote it. I'm confident that you will get a lot more than just one thing.

The Irish M.E. Trust have been immensely helpful. After about 8 years with this condition, I decided something had to change. I hadn't returned to work, and I was mentally and physically not in a good place. I had tried different alternative treatments but needed more, and as good as the medications were, I needed help in other areas.

At this stage I was beat. I knew that if I continued down this road it was not going to do me any good. So, I reached out and asked for help.

The first thing I had to fix was my head. I know I wasn't depressed, but I was definitely down about my situation as I was missing work, had lost my career and all the fun stuff like travel, dancing, skiing, playing football and tennis with my young son.

You will read later how I started to really turn things around with a lady called Louise Keogh. She was amazing. She specialises in Person Centered Therapy. I rewired my thinking and began to come to terms with this condition. The big lesson for me was, if you find yourself in a challenging situation, it's important that you reach out and talk to someone. You need to accept the situation you are in so that you can move on. You are not giving up just adjusting to your new way of handling things. There is no question about it, this, like any other serious condition is not fun and needs to be dealt with on every level. Changes will need to be made to help yourselves. Do what you can to help improve your quality of life and move on the best you can. There is lots of advice in this book. Just take whatever applies to you.

We have our limitations, and we can work around them. I realise it is exceedingly difficult to accept the drastic changes in our lives, and it took me quite a while and a lot of work, but it is possible to accept our situation. It doesn't matter what anyone thinks or says to you, this is real, and change starts with you. It is all about choices and choosing what is best for you.

I know we cannot do a lot of physical things that we did before, but there are low impact physical exercises we can do as long as we pace ourselves e.g. a little stretch or chair yoga. Make sure you get lots of rest and focus on what you can do. I will be going over all this further on in this book. These are just suggestions. It is your choice to do them if you wish. I can tell you that I found them extremely helpful!

Over the years, I have learnt a lot of useful tips and now I am passing them on to you. I use these every day. Not all at once of course, but I pick and choose what I need at any one time. You can improve your quality of life for the better.

You can help yourself. I'm not a doctor but I am someone who has lived with this condition for an awfully long time and what has helped me is in the following pages and it may help you too.

This advice is not limited to people with this condition. It applies to many other debilitating conditions. What I learnt has helped my family enormously in relation to mental strength and general well-being.

Everyone needs to learn how to really look after themselves, so they can be the absolute best version of themselves. We may not have been taught this in school. However, to start with it is particularly important we learn to manage our feelings and emotions.

I started putting this book together a few years ago when I realised how prevalent loneliness, anxiety and mental health issues were.

Everyone from school kids to grandmothers and people with serious illness and working people have problems just trying to find a balance in their lives so they can be happy.

In this book we will look at aspects of life that prove challenging and give suggestions on how to deal with them so you can shake up your life to be more content.

LIFE IS ABOUT THE PEOPLE YOU CHOOSE TO HAVE IN YOUR SPACE, THE PLACES YOU'VE SEEN AND THE MEMORIES YOU MAKE.

MANAGE YOUR EMOTIONS

WE ALL HAVE FLUCTUATING EMOTIONS BUT HAVING A CONDITION LIKE M.E./CFS COMPOUNDS OUR EMOTIONS EVEN MORE.

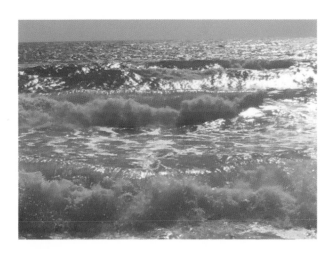

What is M.E./CFS?

I am asked this a lot. I'll start off by saying it is a disabling and complex illness that is quite often misunderstood. It has been described by many sufferers as a bone crushing /overwhelming fatigue that does not improve after rest. I have often had to opt out of going to things with my family as I am completely exhausted from doing little activities. The exhaustion is so strong at times that I do not care if the roof falls down on top of me as there would be no way of moving.

This may sound dramatic to those of you that have not experienced this but believe me it is not an exaggeration.

It is important to learn to handle your emotions and feelings and understand what is going on as the waves can be quite strong. Here are a few things that helped me.

What are feelings?

They are mental experiences of body states which arise as the brain interprets emotions, it's the body's responses to external stimuli i.e., feeling overwhelmed when confronted with an aggressive person, or threatened, fearful, excited etc. It all depends on the situation. Emotions play out in the theatre of the body. Feelings are mental associations and reactions to emotions.

You will suffer if you continue to have an emotional reaction to everything that is said to you. Joy and contentment come from sitting back and observing the situation with logic. If words control you that means everyone else can control you. Breathe, take a chill pill, and let things pass. Don't sweat the small stuff.

Managing your emotions is easier said than done, but it is achievable. You will need to take a good look at the different angles involved and then approach it in a way that you are comfortable with.

Breathing

This is an excellent way of managing the emotional highs and lows. A simple technique as Box Breathing, is as follows:
- Breathe in for four seconds – you should feel your tummy expand.
- Hold for four.
- Breathe out for four seconds – your tummy will return to normal.

You will need to be aware of your breath and how you breathe for this exercise and feel the air moving in and out of your nose. Visualise the hairs in your nose hardly moving. This will slow your breath right down and as a result you will become more relaxed. If you start to drift off and thoughts enter your mind, just return to focussing on your breath.

Meditation

Find a comfortable room and either lie on the bed or sit on a chair. You can find lots of relaxing YouTube videos to listen to for twenty minutes. There will be techniques later in the book.

Mindset

During the Covid-19 pandemic, I found I tended to feel really slug-gish from time to time. The last episode lasted about two weeks where I was dragging myself around the place and feeling I had no interest in doing anything. I needed to change things around. I kept telling myself "Come on you can pull out of this". By the end of the two weeks things had not changed so I had to take a different approach. It is es-pecially important to keep an eye on your moods as this way you can alter them before they dip too low. I gave myself something new to focus on that would stimulate me and shake things up a bit. It is ex-tremely easy to dip into a low mood from time to time. Covid-19 was not helping so I had to put on the thinking cap. In the end I made a conscious decision to get a list going to try and motivate myself. The things on the list were small but they woke up the creative side of my brain. This helped a lot. I knew my energy level was down, so I kept the tasks to 10 minutes each. Even dinners were quick but healthy. I increased water to 2 litres a day minimum and went out in the garden at least 2/3 times during the day for 10 minutes. I cut down the sugar and carbohydrates and increased fibre, and protein. Soon enough I noticed a mood change and things started to get on an even keel. My disinterest disappeared and I started to feel better in myself. It is really important to find what works for you.

Every day when you wake up, you have a choice and you can de-cide to be happy or sad, hopeful, or hopeless. The thing is nobody can make you anything, it's completely up to you. The faster you change your mindset the better life is going to be for yourself: "Today I am going to appreciate what is around me"

SLOW AND STEADY WINS THE RACE

Posture

The way you think is important but the way you hold yourself is particularly important as well. If you stand or sit up straight and keep your chin up, you immediately feel better. Add a smile to your face and presto you are on your way to feeling better. It is very hard to feel bad when you're smiling.

Affirmations

Affirmations are simple positive statements declaring specific goals in their completed states. These empowering mantras have a profound effect on the conscious and unconscious mind, leaving you feeling more content and confident in yourself.

Louse Hay is the lady I turned to many years ago when I first learnt about affirmations. I listened to a CD which is now on YouTube called "101 Power Thoughts Louise Hay".

These are a lovely way to change your mindset and build your self-confidence. I put them on my phone, and they pop up throughout the day to reassure me and keep me emotionally balanced.

Set Boundaries

Boundaries keep us safe and set us free. They also show others what we expect from them. We need to let people know what we will or will not tolerate so that they don't diminish our self-worth and cause ourselves upset.

Please see chapter on Boundaries on page 65 for more information.

Do you want to stay the same?

We all know the expression: "Honesty is the best policy"

If you don't want to stay the same, you're going to have to work at it daily. It is worth it as you will find the people around you will start respecting you more. They will sense the changes in you. At first, they may not like it but, they will adjust also. Just stick with it. Know what you want and go for it.

My suggestion would be to start eliminating feelings from your life like anger, regret, worry, resentment, guilt, and forget about the blame game as that never works out well.

Journalling is a wonderful habit. It's like having a silent friend there whenever you need them, day, or night. Jot down whatever it is you need to figure out. Make it your friend, name it if you want. Go to it when you need to clear out your thoughts. It helps keep you focussed. Have a notebook by your bed. You can also log what you like and what you don't like and change things one at a time. Try not to take on too much as you will be at risk of getting fatigued and overwhelmed.

If you don't manage your emotions, it will cause many problems with your body. Here are a few points to show the impact on your body and thus the importance of keeping your emotions in check:

Shoulder Tension = Burdens and responsibilities
Neck Tension = Fear and repressed self-expression
Upper Back = Grief, sorrow, and sadness
Middle Back = Insecurity and powerlessness
Lower Back = Guilt, shame, and unworthiness
Stomach = Inability to process emotions.
Lungs = Loss

I had to adjust my view on the world. It wasn't doing me any favours worrying and fretting over things that were going on around me that I have no control over.

Try this

Be aware of your surroundings and how they impact on your life. What you do. How it makes you feel. How you dress. Take a good look.
Ask yourself:
"How do I feel when I wear this particular outfit"?
"How does this colour make me feel. Would another one be better"?
Follow your gut and when you wear something that makes you smile and feel confident, go for it. Same goes for other areas of your life, just ask yourself,
"What do I need now?" "How does this make me feel?"

Love the way you love

The way you love someone and how you see people really make a difference. There is good in everyone. How you talk to yourself and others has an impact. You can be unpleasant or comforting in your tone. It costs nothing to be nice, but it makes the world of difference. Your body will thank you in the long run as negativity can have a detrimental effect on you. All those negative vibes are damaging your organs and your health. Be aware of how you treat people. Your smile can change someone's day so wear it. Your personality can lift others so own it, don't hold back.

Be your true self. Enjoy everything you do; from the cup of tea you drink, to the sheets you sleep in at night. Be grateful for every breath you take and every good and bad thing in your life as the bad teaches you and we learn. Be aware of how you feel throughout the day and use the tips and tricks you will learn in this book to alter those feelings to your benefit.

Traffic light system

I use the traffic lights system to gauge my emotions:

Green   You're fine, nice, and calm
Orange You're starting to head for trouble
Red   Logic and everything else flies out the window

The idea of this is to try and stay in the green ideally. When you notice yourself at the orange state take actions straight away.

Three ways to relieve stress are:
1. Breathing.
2. Meditation.
3. Visualisation.

Now make your own list
1.
2.
3.

Being negative only makes the journey more challenging. You may be given a lemon, but you can always make lemonade.

BE YOURSELF UNAPOLOGETICALLY. LET PEOPLE SEE
THE REAL YOU. IT TAKES A LOT LESS ENERGY. IT'S OK TO
HAVE IMPERFECTIONS, FLAWS, AND INDIVIDUAL QUIRKS,
THAT'S WHAT MAKES YOU UNIQUE AND BEAUTIFUL. YOU
ARE MAGICAL JUST THE WAY YOU ARE!

FEAR

BEWARE OF DREAM, PASSION, AND VISION KILLERS!

Here is what I know for sure. High vibes always overcome low vibes, so managing your thoughts is first and foremost.
You become what you believe to be true, so be aware of what is going through your mind and choose wisely.

Remember: Believe that anything is possible!
You have everything you need within you to become whatever you want. I realise we have limitations, and everybody is different but none of us know what is ahead of us, so anything is possible.

You can manifest miracles; it has happened before so there is no reason it can't happen again.

Gratitude has an amazing effect on the body.
Fear will squash all your dreams. Thinking in the future will fuel fear so try as much as possible to be present.

Start by eliminating, judgement, anger, regret, worry, resentment, guilt, and blame. Then watch your health and life improve.

Here are a few tips on how to deal with fear:
Fear happens when you think you must figure everything out at once. You don't!

Breathe.

Take a moment for yourself. You've got this!

Just take it step by step.

Is there a fear of something holding you back in life? Fear of failure or fear of making yourself more unwell? I can understand this as I felt it for a long time and it's extremely easy to overdo things. Pacing yourself will help a lot. I know it takes discipline but if it helps keep the wolf from the door it is worth it. We all get afraid but how we handle fear will result in how fast we get through it.

Try to look at the situation from different angles and see if you can work something out by compromising a little on your plans. Do what suits you at any particular time. Don't be pressured to stay longer at a party or do anything that makes you uncomfortable like staying in anyone's company any longer than you want to. If you let fear hold you back, you will end up extremely limited and restricted. This is where journalling is excellent as you can write down the situation or challenge and work it out on paper.

Even though as teenagers and adults we no longer fear monsters under our beds, fears persist in our lives in subtle forms.

Fear of failure.

Fear of regret.

Fear of the future.

Fear is an emotion and like other emotions it can be managed. Don't let fear stop you. Take things at your own pace and keep it manageable. Keep moving forward. Life will present different challenges for you and you are capable of handling whatever comes your way. Fear is the most destructive thing. It destroys you, puts people in hospital, ages you, paralyses you and holds you back. There are no benefits to giving up. You are going to make mistakes. You're not perfect and that's ok.

NOBODY IS PERFECT.
WE MAKE MISTAKES.
WE SAY THE WRONG THING.
WE DO WRONG THINGS.
WE FALL. WE GET UP. WE LEARN.
WE GROW. WE MOVE ON. WE LIVE.

Remember: You can live your dreams or live your fears, it's your choice.

Face your fears again and again and again otherwise you will not grow. Dream about what you want. I visualise myself with better health all the time. Positive Self Talk is enormously powerful.

Acknowledge your fears and embrace them but don't let them paralyse you.

It's ok to have fears. Take the necessary precautions and move forward. Remember, baby steps, one at a time and if you take two steps forward and four steps back, that's ok because you are strong enough to start again. I have started over so many times. I rest up and start again because I believed always and still do, that I will get through this.

I have never met a person with this condition who isn't a fighter. The will to get better and move on is in us.

What you resist will persist. Acceptance was a huge breakthrough for me. It was quite challenging but once I got my head around the fact that I was not giving up, just saying goodbye to the old me and embracing the new me, things shifted. You will be the better for this as it's part of the recovery process and the main aim is to get a better quality of life. It's important to point out that you are not giving in. You are focussing your energy on the things that matter and that will help you.

Don't stop living your dreams. Always hold on to them. Don't surrender to your fears. I use visualisation to take me to the places I can't go. The great thing is the mind doesn't know the difference.

See how far you have come. Be proud of yourself. One day, you can look at someone straight in the eye and say, "I lived through it and it made me who I am today"

You will feel mentally stronger if you do the exercises that are in this book and over time you will be able to do a bit more and be more content. I do things in 5,10,15, or 20 minute, intervals, whatever I'm able for in the day. It differs day to day and that's our reality but that's ok and if it takes me five times longer to get small jobs done, i.e., tidy my room, I get there in the end by pacing it out in a time frame that suits me. You can do the same by just asking yourself, "What do I need to get done here?" and "how long can I spend on this today?" If it's not finished just come back each day for a short time that suits you and before you know it, the task will be completed.

TRUST YOURSELF, DO NOT FEAR.
AS YOU KNOW MORE THAN YOU THINK YOU DO.

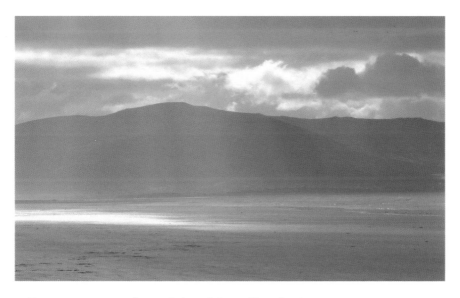

Fear can stop us from doing things if we let it.

I was on a plane once, not a very big one, maybe an eight-seater. I was quite young, about fourteen years old. After the plane was taking off, all was well, but about twenty minutes into the flight things started to take a dramatic turn for the worse. We hit a storm and the small aircraft was being challenged to its limits. Everyone on board was ter-rified. Now you'd think after going through something like that you'd never fly again, and the fear would completely put you off. It didn't because my mum reassured me that everything would be fine, and it was.

Now, this thankfully taught me a valuable lesson which I did not realise until later. In life you can't think of two things at once so if you distract yourself from the present situation and substitute it with something else you can get through what is facing you.

I have used this tactic more than once, and it works beautifully. One time was when my husband, son and I decided to go on a boat trip while on holidays and it was going well until we hit bad weather and had to turn around with great difficulty and head back to shore. Everyone on the boat was crying and getting sick and my young son was getting quite pale so I automatically changed my tune and started to say things like, "isn't this exciting, this is some pirate ship, what an adventure we are on today" and so on and in the end, he couldn't hear anyone but me and we started making up all these stories about adventures on boats. When we eventually got to shore, they handed our money back to us as we left. We didn't even have to ask! That will tell you how scary the ride was but while everyone else had angry faces my son got off the boat that day with a smile and afterwards when he had gone to bed my husband and I thanked our lucky stars.

Fear about the future is very understandable, but the truth is none of us have any control over what happens tomorrow so don't waste your time worrying as everything will take care of itself. Take things as they come and handle each situation as it arises.

The uncertainty of a particular situation you're in, can throw you into a spin. To think clearly you will need to take a deep breath and take things one step at a time. Write down a plan of action and keep it simple. You can do this daily and weekly. Space everything out into manageable chunks.

We can't always see whether we'll fail or succeed, whether we'll be completely satisfied with our choices, or what the future will hold. We just have to trust that we will do the right thing at the time. Worrying will not improve the situation.

With time you will learn to let go of your uncertainty as you will realise that nothing is guaranteed and not everything is completely fixed. You must take a chance and hope for the best. Things will change and not always for the worse. Nothing is static. If you take that step towards what you fear, you could be surprised at how great the results are and that you had nothing to fear all along. You will not know until you take the first step and then the next, and so on.

Weigh up all your options and see what they look like. Don't overthink things too much. I'm a terror for overthinking. I have improved a lot and so can you. Overthinking will send your head into a spin. Keep things simple.

M A M

M = Motivation, what makes you want to do things or overcome your obstacles.

A = Attention, pay attention to what excites you and gets you motivated and use it. This will put a smile on your face.

M= Mechanics, are the tools you use to get what you want.

Before you go anywhere or do anything, remind yourself that you are good enough to achieve it and that you deserve it. It is especially important to believe in yourself. If you have a fear about something, name it and come up with a plan to get through it.

First look at your motivation, i.e. how will I feel if I do this? Find your "why" and feel it and let that motivate you. Plan what tools you are going to use to achieve it.

For example, I use breathing to relax and ground myself. You can choose whatever works for you.

Remind yourself every hour to take three breaths. I find the app "Chimes", useful. It literally "chimes" every hour and this reminds me to check my breathing and make sure I'm grounded.

It only takes a couple of seconds to do the following breathing exercise and it is extremely effective. I use it sometimes before phone conversations. I just put one hand on my tummy and one hand on my chest. Then I take a breath in through my nose for a count of four. As I breathe in, my tummy expands but my chest doesn't move up. It is important to focus on the tummy. Then I hold for a moment, and when I breathe out through my nose for a count of six, I feel myself releasing all my tension and becoming grounded. I notice a real difference. Even the tone I use is more relaxed and I think more clearly.

FEAR IS A STATE OF MIND THAT CAN BE CHANGED AT ANY TIME, SO LET GO A LITTLE AND BE KIND TO YOURSELF AND OTHERS. YOU WILL FIND LIFE A LOT EASIER.

ANXIETY

"YOU MAY NOT FEEL STRONG BUT
IN SOMEONE ELSE'S EYE'S
YOU ARE THEIR STRENGTH"

You may ask yourself: 'What exactly is anxiety'?
Here are a few things to look at to clarify how you may feel with anxiety:

Not able to think straight.
Getting confused.
Feeling lonely.
Not in the present.
Your mind wandering to past and future.
Not able to think straight.
Getting confused.
Feeling lonely
Not in the present
Your mind wandering to past and future.

Anxiety can affect events and activities as you don't feel comfortable in particular situations. You are not always tuned in or present. You notice yourself drifting off and come back not knowing what the person you are talking to is saying. You have completely zoned out.

Anxiety is present when you are noticing the following:
- Irrational behaviour.
- Mood swings.
- Constant worrying over the smallest of things.
- People pleasing too much.
- Fear.
- Thinking something bad is going to happen.
- Feeling unable and too afraid to speak up.
- Self-criticising your every move.
- Not wanting to come across as stupid.
- Thinking you must be perfect to avoid judgement.
- Feeling like you must overachieve to be considered intelligent.
- Believing everyone is judging you and talking behind your back.
- Feeling you are not good enough.

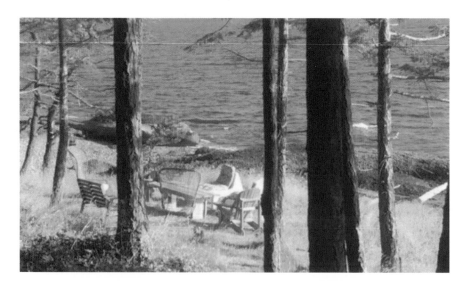

Have you noticed yourself experiencing any of the above?
You can tick the ones you experience as it is good to be aware. Next ask yourself, "what can I do to change these?" and come up with an action plan.

How anxiety affects the body and mind

Here are a few examples:

Physical and Emotional Behaviour changes.

- Feeling sick.
- Overwhelmed.
- Smoking extra.
- Tension.
- Confused & Flustered.
- Increased intake of Drink/Drugs.
- Butterflies in your tummy.
- Increased anger.
- Sadness & Frustration.
- Withdrawn from people.
- Panic Attacks.
- Feeling Irritable.
- Eating habits change.
- Eating Disorders.
- Lack of Sleep/Exhaustion.
- Helplessness.
- Lack of self-confidence, never feeling comfortable in others company.
- Restlessness.
- Sickness.
- Mentally drained
- Shouting a lot more.
- Fearful.
- Aches & Pains.
- Lowered immunity.
- Argumentative.
- Overthinking & analysing everything.

Do you recognise any of the above in yourself? Take a moment to read over them again. It doesn't matter if the list seems remarkably familiar to you as it is good to be aware of these things. You can now start to alter your anxiety. You will feel much better, it takes a little work but it's worth it.

Try this:

Slowing down your heart rate by using the breathing technique we discussed earlier. You can alter it slightly by breathing in for a count of 4 seconds, hold for 2 and exhale for 6 seconds. This will activate the vagus nerve which is the healing nerve.

Here are a couple of things I recommend you to do every morning. You can make these a routine if you like. They only take a minute and help to make you feel better. You can do these when you are brushing your teeth first thing in the morning as it will give you a good state of mind for the day ahead.

1. Name five things you are grateful for.
2. Name one thing you love about yourself.
3. What is your main intention for today?
4. How do you want to feel today?

When you have answered these questions stand up tall and put your hands on your hips. Put your shoulders back and chin up, look yourself in the eye, in the mirror and say "I am enough, and I will always be enough! I've got this!" Repeat this mantra 3 times and really mean it and feel it! Don't forget to smile. Now you are ready to face the day ahead. Next, put on uplifting music and have a delicious breakfast.

Nobody is right all the time

Lose the fear of being wrong. Mistakes are good, as you learn from them and grow. Don't beat yourself up about it. Self-Talk can be your best friend or your greatest downfall. Try working on positive self-esteem and confidence.

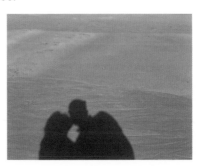

Know that you are loved.

It is human to be imperfectly perfect. To grow and have successes, you must make some mistakes along the way. I have made many and have lived to laugh about them. Each day is a new day to live and learn.

"ONCE YOU CHANGE THE WAY YOU LOOK AT EVERYTHING, THINGS WILL ALTER"

It is especially important to be open minded and listen to other people's point of view. This way we can learn things and view them from a different perspective. When you are trying something new it is always good to get all the information regarding the change you are wishing to make.

I decided to give up dairy and meat a few years ago. I talked to a lot of people and researched the benefits to my health. As it turned out there were huge benefits to my health as I was intolerant to dairy and had asthma. The advantage to giving up meat was it was easier to digest other foods. I investigated doing it properly and ended up loving it and never looked back.

We need to be open and listening to all sides. Nobody is wrong or right we just see things from a different angle. Be kind in your approach to others. This will benefit both you and them. Save your energy. Take a softer approach. It's not always important to be right as we all have a different point of view.

Affirmations for letting go

It's good to shed the past and say goodbye. I use the following:
Repeat as often as you can

"TODAY I EMBRACE THE MEMORY OF MY PAST AND I AM GRATEFUL FOR ALL THAT LIFE HAS GIVEN ME." "I ACKNOWLEDGE THAT I DID THE BEST I COULD AT THE TIME, AND NOW I AM READY TO LET GO. I AM CLEAR ABOUT MY PATH AHEAD AND LOOK FORWARD TO GOOD

TIMES." "I WELCOME WITH OPEN ARMS ALL THE ABUNDANCES THAT ARE COMING AND LOOK FORWARD TO ALL THE WONDERFUL HAPPY SURPRISES THAT ARE ON THE WAY TO ME." "I TREAT OTHERS AS I WISH TO BE TREATED." "I AM GRATEFUL FOR ALL THE BLESSINGS IN MY LIFE." "I AM GETTING STRONGER AND STRONGER EVERY DAY."

Finding the right support

So many people come to me saying their doctor doesn't understand what they are going through. I usually suggest getting another doctor and keep going until they get one that supports them and their needs. There is plenty of help there, but you have to go and find it. I am blessed with my doctor as he supports and understands what I am going through.

Whatever your circumstances, there is a solution. You may have to adjust your way of life and your thought process along the way.

Ask yourself "What am I willing to do to improve my situation?" I had issues with my digestive system and ended up going for a scan. The doctor talked to me afterwards and said there was nothing seriously wrong as it was just a case of eating foods that didn't agree with me. His advice was "If a food doesn't agree with you, stop eating it" So I started making a note of the foods I was eating in a notebook and eliminated the ones that triggered an upset tummy. I also introduced Digestive Enzymes which I found fantastic. I read about them on Healthline.com. PubMed is a highly respected database from the National Institute of Health and is a great resource for information.

If your digestive system is not working and you suffer from a lot of tummy issues, stop eating food that disagrees with you. Hopefully, this will help.

Address the issues that apply to you one by one, and you will start to have a better quality of life.

Remember:

Life is like a boomerang. What you send out, comes back. What you sow, you reap. What you give, you get. What you see in others, exists in you. Treat others like you want to be treated. That way life gets easier.

Every situation in life is temporary. So, when life is good, make sure you enjoy and receive it fully. And when life is not good remember that it will not last forever, and better days are on the way.

THOUGHTS

WITH THOUGHTS YOU WANT TO KEEP THE GOOD ONES AND GET RID OF THE REST ASAP

Apparently, we have 2,056,000 thoughts a day! A large portion of these are negative.

Why do we overthink things?
This helped me simplify:
If you are:

Missing somebody	Call
Wanna meet up	Invite
Wanna be understood	Explain
Don't like something	Say it
Have a question	Ask
Like something	State it
Love someone.	Tell them.

It doesn't get easier than that.

Thoughts
Our circumstances lead to our thoughts
Our thoughts cause our feelings

Our feelings drive our actions
And our actions create our results
I found it helped to understand how thoughts worked.
Thoughts can be divided into three categories. They are as follows:

Rational thoughts
These are thoughts that make sense.
We make decisions based on logic and past events.
In order to have rational thoughts we need to deal with suppressed emotions.

Wise thoughts
Balanced, not too high, or too low. On an even keel.
Honour emotions and strive to act rationally.
We need to be mindful, aware, and present as much as possible.

Emotional thoughts
These are thoughts that feel right. Listen to your gut. It could save your life.
Emotions can be reactive and defensive. It is important to be aware of your emotions and try not to overreact to situations. Try to breathe and count to 3, or 10 if required.

The emotional side can often be opposite to the rational side. Do you go with the heart or the mind? I say follow your gut, but you can decide for yourself. I have found when I don't listen to my gut it usually comes back at me, so now I try to listen to my gut all the time. If I get a strong feeling in my gut, I follow it. I've learnt to trust my gut through practicing relaxation and meditation.

Be suave
B = Believe in yourself. You've got this.
E = Exercise (go over your plan to get you through your obstacles)
S = Say what you plan to say in a situation, whatever that may be, i.e. handling difficult people or remembering names etc.
U = Use people's name if you have problems remembering them

A = Ask. Don't be afraid to ask people to repeat what they say if you didn't catch it or you don't remember their names.

V = Visualise. This will help you remember things.

E = Enjoy Life.

WHAT YOU HEAR YOU FORGET WHAT YOU SEE YOU
REMEMBER WHAT YOU DO YOU UNDERSTAND
T. Harv Eker

YOUR ANXIETY
IS LYING TO YOU.
YOU ARE LOVED.
YOU ARE STRONG.
YOU ARE GOING TO BE OKAY.
BELIEVE IN YOURSELF.
THIS TOO SHALL PASS.

There is a lot of truth in the expression,
"WHAT YOU THINK ABOUT, YOU BRING ABOUT"
Be very careful with your thoughts and words. Your brain does what it's told. If you go around saying "I'm stupid for doing that" or "this job is killing me" or "this kid will be the death of me," the brain takes it all literally. It views everything as a command. It doesn't have a sense of humour.

Take a different approach and you will notice things start looking a whole lot better. Try "My kid is age appropriate" or "My job is challenging but I love it" or "I am going to pay more attention to what I am doing."

It will take being more aware of your thoughts and conversations at first, but it will become second nature in the end.

Try this:

Place small red circular stickers in places you'll see them, for example, your mirror, fridge, car. They will remind you to stop and change the thoughts.

Speak of what you want not what you don't want.

Having conflicting thoughts e.g. eating a slice of cake and then feeling guilty, saying to yourself "I shouldn't be eating this but…". Just decide, choose to eat it, or don't eat it but accept what you decide and move on. If you eat it, enjoy it without the guilt. Anything you choose to do, enjoy and be content that you chose it. It's in your power to choose what is best for you so do it whole heartedly.

Decide, there is nowhere you'd rather be than right here doing whatever it is you choose to do. Be in the here and now. Be in the moment with what you are doing right now.

Remember:

Think about what you want, say it, and go for it. Aim high!

Thoughts and beliefs will limit you so avoid negative ones. If someone puts you down, you'd feel bad, wouldn't you? So why do you do it to yourself? This is just a bad habit you can change. You have the choice to believe whatever you want, so have fun with it. With thoughts you have a physical and emotional response within your body, so be kind to yourself and choose carefully how you think.

There will always be ups and downs, good times and bad, losses and gains. Life is about learning lessons and showing love in the process and growing. Choose to be happy no matter what the day throws at you.

The brain only knows the positive and the negative. The positive will lead to good thoughts and vibes in the body which will end with good health. The negative unfortunately is the opposite and will therefore lead to unhappiness and ill health.

The good news is we have the power to choose.

WHEN I REALISE THAT I AM HAVING A NEGATIVE THOUGHT, I REPLACE IT WITH AT LEAST 3 POSITIVE ONES.

Procrastination

Don't let procrastination get in your way. If it's important enough you will do it. You won't even think about it. You'll just spring into action. Things we love to do are always high on our priority list. If something is high on your priority list, you won't put them off. It's things that are low on your priority list you need to be aware of and not procrastinate on. Make a list of what it is you need to do. Then break it up into manageable sections and do twenty minutes a day. This will reduce some of the stress and anxiety you feel, and you will be more likely to do the task.

I tell myself that I only have to work for two minutes on the task today. Then I can continue another day. If that still doesn't get me going, I just ask myself for 1 minute of work. I can do that one minute of work in a very relaxed pace. I always do more because my enthusiasm grows, and momentum builds.

No matter how small a task, tick it off the list when it's done. It feels great. What I do is tell myself "If I do this then I can have that afterwards. Example, when I work on this book for x amount of time, I can have a mug of my favourite tea and a square of dark chocolate. Treat yourself after each achievement. It doesn't have to be food all the time as we don't want you running up the scales now, do we? So maybe record your favourite show and watch it when you're finished your task; or call a friend. You make the rules so have fun with it.

Make the start as easy and light as you can. Be kind to yourself in this way and you'll be amazed at how much you can get started and done.

Name 3 areas in your life where you have been procrastinating:
1.
2.
3.

Now ask yourself "How can I get things moving in these areas"
1.
2.
3.

VISUALISATION

VISUALISE WHAT YOU WANT

Try visualising a beautiful turquoise wave for me and see the way it curves. You have the tip of the wave before it breaks and then you have it nice and flat after it has landed on the shore. Our emotions are remarkably similar. Now if you are aware of this in your body you can manage the waves of emotions and calm them through using different techniques.

If you want something:

- Feel it and be there, in the moment.
- Want it
- Get a clear picture in your head.
- Now plan how you are going to get there step by step.

Start today!

I have found Visualisation a fantastic tool that I use regularly. I can't visit all the places I want so I go in my mind whenever I want. I often take a trip in my imagination to different parts of the globe and it always leaves me with a smile on my face. If my mood is dipping it is an instant break away from my unpleasant thoughts. It is definitely one of my most rewarding tools that I use, and it has helped me cope through many turbulent times.

DECIDE AND CHOOSE WHO
AND WHAT YOU WANT TO BE OR
WHERE YOU WANT TO GO. THEN TAKE ACTION.

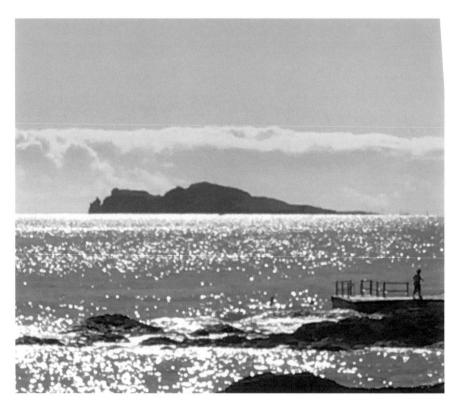

Get comfortable

Find a comfortable place to sit where you can relax in peace and quiet. Here is an exercise to show you the power of visualisation, and the power it has on your overall feelings.

Start with this breathing exercise

The aim with breathing exercises is to slow everything down. They help to lower the heart rate and will put you in a more relaxed state of mind. This will also benefit the Vagus Nerve, which is the main nerve that goes through your body. It interacts with the heart, lungs, and digestive tract. It plays a vital role in your wellbeing. See Medd.org-vagus-nerve stimulation and its many benefits – Mindd Foundation and Harvard Programme in Neuroscience PhD Programme.

Get yourself nice and comfortable and place your two feet flat on the ground. You can remove your shoes if you like. This will help to ground you. Bring your attention into the inside of your body. I usually start by placing a hand on my tummy. This helps me to focus on a particular part of my body. Now, take a nice big breath in for the count of 4 and hold for 2, and exhale for 6. It is always good to make the exhale longer than the inhale as it benefits the body more.

Do this 4 times. You will feel much more relaxed. This is very quick to do and if you can repeat it a few times a day or any time you're feeling stress, anxiety or you just want to gather your thoughts, it will help you immensely.

Now visualise your favourite cake e.g. chocolate with hot sauce and add some ice cream if you wish. "Does this make you feel good?"

Now visualise a puppy out in the cold on a stormy night. It is pouring rain and he hasn't been fed for a few days. "Does this make you feel bad?"

Now to get you back to feeling good again. Picture a beautiful beach, by a 5-star hotel with unlimited food and drink. Everybody is friendly. Presto, you feel good again, and I bet there is a smile on your face. You can change your feelings through visualisation, it's very easy.

Life is about figuring out what you want and need and mapping a plan to get it. No matter how small or big your dream is, make a start and work towards it.

Look at your own situation and decide what you're going to do about it. It could be anything from dealing with difficult people in your life to just feeling better in yourself. Make a plan and head for the results you desire.

3D visualisation
This is where you visualise, but you go one step further. Imagine

yourself sitting on a comfortable chair and you are feeling very relaxed. Your eyes are closed. Now visualise yourself standing up and walking into the kitchen. Have a good look around and see everything you usually would see in there and name them e.g. the cooker, the cupboards etc. Now go to where the fridge is and open it. What do you see? Pick something up and feel it. We will use a piece of fresh cut lemon as an example. Now bite into the lemon. Can you taste it? I bet you can. Is your mouth becoming full of juices just at the thought of it? That is 3D visualisation. When you can taste things and feel them, then you're there. It's like magic.

DECIDE WHAT YOU WANT TO HAPPEN AND THEN: CONTROL THE CONTROLLABLES

You always have a choice, so choose wisely. You can't control everything, so don't drive yourself crazy trying to. Take a good look at what is going on and control what you can e.g., your attitude, what you eat, how much you sleep, who you hang out with, how much negativity you are prepared to take from your friends and family.

Focus
Be present and aware. Ground yourself. Breathe and stay calm. Focus on one thing at a time so you don't get flustered as this will cause irritation and annoyance.

Plan
What are you going to do about the situation you are in? Write it down. Visualise what you want.

Take action
Start putting your plan in motion. Take the first step.

Remember:
Dreams are Possible! Just ask Lady Gaga or Barack Obama who came from nothing along with a lot of other famous people. Note that

I am not saying you'll be famous. Make a start at mastering each day to suit yourself. Get little things done and tick them off your list. Who knows where it will lead.

People have opinions and that's ok but they're not always right. We can choose to differ. Don't let one person's opinion of you put you off your dream. If you want something bad enough you will find a way to get it. Anything is possible.

Be in charge of your destiny. Surround yourself with people that believe in you and share your views. Don't waste your time on negative people as they will only bring you down and you are on your way up.

Believe you can do it. Find a way around your obstacles.

Believe you can change for the better. The aim here is to improve your quality of life. You can improve your quality of life! No matter how small your dream, go for it. What is the worst that can happen? You end up exactly where you are right now? So at least you tried. If you don't make a start you will never know. Most of the time you benefit somewhat as you will always learn something from what you try. There are lots of changes you can make to improve your life. Sit with it and ask yourself "Where do I want to start?".

I started with relaxation and calming everything down. Then I went onto food and dealing with migraines. Read through this book and take notes. Adjust habits that will benefit you. This is a book you can read back over to refresh different areas.

Don't let your limitations, whatever they may be, stop you.

Start small and work your way through whatever your wish is. That way it has the hope of becoming reality.

YOU CAN DO THIS,
FACE LIFE HEAD ON,
AT YOUR OWN PACE.
GO STEP BY STEP.
YOU WILL BE JUST FINE.

Try this:

Do you ever find yourself in bed trying to get to sleep and just can't seem to clear your mind of all the thoughts from the day? Conversations you've had. Thinking of what you should have said or done. Do you keep going over and over them again until you realise it is late into the night?

Here is a trick I use to sort that out.

It's called gone, gone

Imagine you are in a classroom and there is a whiteboard on the wall. It is full of all the stuff that is running around in your head and keeping you from getting to sleep. Pick up the eraser and wipe all that stuff off until the board is back to white again and everything is Gone, Gone. Now you can reassure yourself that there is nothing you can do about anything at this time of night. You can get a good night's sleep and face the day tomorrow with a fresh perspective and a clear mind.

You see the past is the past and it is gone forever. There is only one way forward so cut the past free and get some sleep.

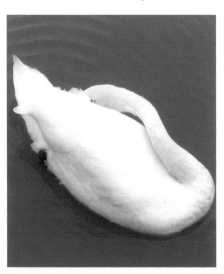

BE SELECTIVE IN YOUR BATTLES. IS IT REALLY WORTH
GETTING INTO SOME CONVERSATIONS?
SOMETIMES YOU JUST HAVE TO LET IT GO

GETTING TO KNOW YOURSELF:

LOVE AND LAUGHTER IS WHAT MAKES EVERY DAY WORTHWHILE

A lot of you have pets. The love an animal gives you is like gold dust. It is so pure and unconditional. I often say if humans could have the heart of a dog what a wonderful world it would be.

How well do you know yourself?
Get to know yourself by writing down your strengths and weaknesses.
Try this:
One really good way to get to know yourself is to get a plain sheet of paper and a pen. Draw a circle.
This can be your head. You can put in eyes, a nose and a mouth if you wish. Above your head put different size clouds. Start with five big ones and five smaller ones with a few medium ones. Each one represents a different trait. The size of the cloud represents the size of the strength or weakness e.g. anger may be a big issue for you that you may need to work on. Place this in a big cloud. When you have worked to reduce your anger, you can replace it in a smaller cloud later. Now take a good look at yourself and decide what your personal traits are i.e. good personality, friendly, happy, stubborn, fearful, over-cautious,

bad at communicating with friends, selfish at times, inquisitive etc. Also, look at time spent with family, friends, time in nature, days out, holidays, and so on. Take a close look at all aspects of your life, good and not so good. This way you get a clear picture. You can have as many clouds as you like. Give yourself plenty of room.

Now put the most significant traits in the big clouds and put the insignificant ones in the small clouds. And others that you're not sure of go in the medium clouds.

When you are finished, stand back, and take a good look at what you put where and adjust if needed.

This will give you a clear picture of all the aspects of your life. Be honest with yourself. No one will see this only you. Have fun with it.

Next, choose what you want to work on. Some clouds you will want to increase and bring more of into your life e.g. happiness. Others, like anger you'll want to reduce down to extra small clouds, as they are not serving you at all.

The exercise is to cut out the weaknesses as much as possible and increase the strengths.

Now we are all human so things like anger and frustration, will pop up but, if we are more conscious of our actions, we can stop them quicker.

Same goes for the medium clouds. It's all about tweaking the clouds to the size you want. This way the characteristics you like, get bigger and bigger and take over.

It's time to start making conscious decisions and adjusting your focus on what you want. Watch how things change. Watch and see how what is good in you grows.

Did you ever notice that when someone tells you about a certain type of car, all you notice when you're out is that type of car? Suddenly you are seeing it everywhere. I was dropping my car to be scrapped last year and when I was returning home, I spotted 3 cars of the same colour and year. That was very unusual as it was fifteen years old, so I very rarely saw more than one a week let alone 3 in one day. The point I'm making here is you attract what you're thinking about. Some call it, coincidences. Others, the law of attraction. The bottom line is that conscious decisions can improve your life.

Your quality of life can improve day by day. In time you will have all your good traits in large bubbles and your unwanted ones will not be a problem anymore.

When you do this the first time you may be pleasantly surprised. You will discover things about yourself that you had forgotten about.

It will shine a light on everything and make it clearer so you can put your attention where it is needed. I really found this exercise greatly beneficial. I used to get very lonely but now it's very rare that this happens. I started looking at low impact activities that I could start introducing that I enjoyed. I rejigged my focus and put my energy into the areas that brought me joy and contentment. I chose things like photography, writing, meditation, just going out in the garden more looking at the plants, pruning the roses, reading, etc. When I increase these and decreased things like worry, fretting, anger, judgement, frustration etc, things started to improve a lot for me. You see a lot of this internal stuff can be very damaging so the more we get a handle on it the better our lives will be.

Change won't happen overnight, just take it nice and slow, be patient and kind with yourself.

IT DOESN'T MATTER HOW SLOW YOU GO AS LONG AS YOU BELIEVE IN YOURSELF AND KEEP FOCUSSED ON THE END RESULT...STEP BY STEP YOU WILL GET THERE!

How to take action

Having a plan is only half the job. I believe that the most important thing is simply to act. It's not easy and you often get stuck. Focus and ask yourself, "what do I want?" and "what do I need to do next to get this done?" You can visualise a bridge. You are on one side and your completed task is on the other. Make a list of what you can do to reach your goals. To cross over the bridge, you will need to take action, one step at a time and you will get there. It can be a simple task like clearing your wardrobe out, or getting your filing done or to stop reacting to triggers etc.

I tended to overthink things and then never got things done. It was only when I started making lists that this changed, and I overcame this trait. I adjusted my habits, and that helped me to get tasks completed.

Prioritise

Make a list of your top priorities and pick what needs to be dealt with first.

What is the most important thing on the list that needs to be dealt with? You won't need much motivation for this one as it is a must.

When that first and most important task is done, you tick it off your list, and you instantly feel better. Then move onto the next item.

It's really motivating, and a good feeling comes over you as each achievement has been reached.

Take responsibility for your actions:

Own what you decide to do. Be proud and stand tall. Enjoy doing it and be in the moment. Don't waste your time with trying to impress people or be a people pleaser. This takes up too much of your time and energy. Just be yourself and do what you want at your own pace.

To get anything done you need to make a list and plan what actions you are going to take.

Things will not always turn out how you plan but that's okay. You can't control the results of all your actions. You also can't predict how someone will react to what you say or do. Don't worry too much about that as you can tweak things and learn from your mistakes. Nobody is perfect.

It is especially important to enjoy what you do, as you will be far more motivated and achieve a lot more that way.

Act on tasks you want to get done. It is so much easier when you break up the task into small pieces. It is less overwhelming that way.

Say you want to try a new food recipe. It can look really complicated at first but when you go step by step you will eventually get to the end and find it really wasn't that bad.

STEP BY STEP, DAY BY DAY, NICE AND EASY ALL THE WAY.

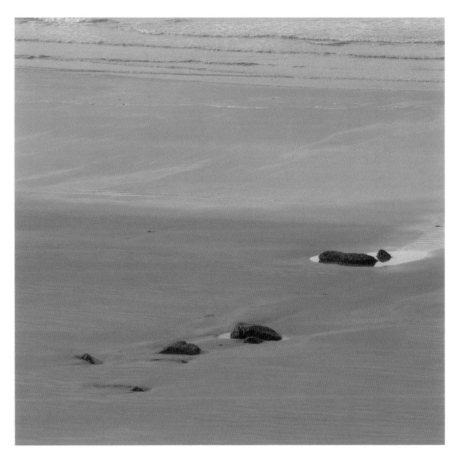

The following came out of a Diary for Busy Women 2020 and I thought it was lovely.

The Empty Chair
I forgot to love myself today when pain was all around.
I forgot to pay attention to the courage I had found.
I forgot that many love me, much more than I can tell.
I forgot that this is a time for peace and love as well.
I forgot that sadness on one day doesn't count for all the years.
I forgot how much a simple hug could allay so many fears.

I forgot that on my forehead once a loving kiss was placed.
I forgot that there are many loves, and each one has its place.
I forgot to love myself today and saw the flowers there.
I forgot it was a special thing to be in someone's prayer.
I forgot that I am blessed with life and may go too quick.
I forgot that in life's moments and beauty doesn't last.
I forgot that years could pass us by so amazingly fast.
I forgot the words of poems and love-songs we would sing.
And remembered that friendship, love, and gratitude is truly everything.
Unknown

ACCEPTANCE

Acceptance is the area I found the most difficult to deal with. We are not always going to like what we are doing. Not everything is fun. It takes time to get your head around things sometimes and once you do, you can move on and adjust.

Like anyone living with a chronic illness, I realised after several years there is only so much that mainstream medicine could do. It was time for me to look further to see if there was anything else out there that would help my situation. I realised that things like diet, exercise, and lifestyle were my responsibility not the medics. When I say exercise, I'm talking about a nice leisurely walk in the fresh air for short periods of time that I was able for. Everybody differs in this area. It all depends on the severity of your condition and your attitude.

Then I started to investigate complementary medicine. These are treatments that are used along with standard medical treatments but are not considered to be standard treatments, e.g. acupuncture. I asked around and found someone with a good reputation who had dealt with M.E./CFS before.

This is a neurological condition not a psychological one. In 2009, I turned to the Irish M.E. Trust for help. I was feeling very lost and had no vision of where my life was going. I was not dealing with my condition very well. It was starting to get on top of me both physically and mentally. I talked to Declan Carroll of the Irish M.E. Trust. He was very understanding and pointed me in the direction of Louise Keogh, a Person Centred Therapist. She is accredited with IACP and has a BSc in Counselling and Psychotherapy. This helped me to get my thoughts clear in my head as I wanted to sort out my limitations and how to deal with them.

What Louise's work did very well was to help me adjust my thinking and how to live with this condition. She helped me to accept the changes I needed to make. This eased the stress anxiety and frustration caused by not being able to do things. Louise explains below about Person Centred Therapy and how we worked together.

Carl Rogers developed Person-Centred Therapy in the 1940's. My training as a Person-Centred Therapist began in 2006. A Rogerian or Person-Centred Therapist learns to recognise and trust human potential. It provides clients with empathy, congruence, and unconditional positive regard, to facilitate personal growth and change. The therapist avoids directing the course of therapy by following the client's lead whenever possible. The therapist offers support, guidance, and structure so that the client can discover personalised solutions within themselves. My solution may not be their solution.

Nowadays, I consider myself more of an Integrative Therapist whereby I apply different modalities (i.e. Cognitive Behavioural Therapy (CBT) or Solution Focused Therapy etc.) I have gained through training, experience, and best practice, to suit the clients' needs. My role as a therapist with the Irish M.E. Trust started in 2009, whereby I offered support to members who had a diagnosis or suffered from symptoms of M.E./Chronic Fatigue.

It was in 2010 that I received the referral of Sarah from the Irish M.E. Trust. Sarah engaged in phone therapy for a period of one year initially and then reached out for further support in the following years. At the beginning of therapy with a new client it was important that I built a good relationship, provided a safe space where Sarah could be open and honest about her health condition and the impact it was having on her life without feeling judged.

Sarah describes the impact of her illness as a volcano, where she builds and builds and then blows, all this hurt, and frustration just flows out of her like lava:

"I hate telling people I have M.E. or being labelled as depressed". Sarah like most M.E./CFS suffers is grieving the loss of her life, control of her health, being physically active, career, finance, independence, engaging in sport activities and especially social interactions. By acknowledging Sarah's limitations and her individuality within her condition we were able to slowly work toward a new MAP of her life. This being to Manage, Accept and Pace and in time hopefully maintain her learnings, insights, triggers, and limitations to enable a more fulfilled life.

I feel Sarah would agree that we faced many a challenge during the therapeutic process and we even described it with humour as like being in a boxing ring. Fighting to accept the facts, impact and limitations of her diagnoses, denial, resistance, and fear of the future. In Sarah's own words: "M.E. is pissing me off, I have no purpose or time for this illness and can't accept this life".

After seven months of weekly therapy, Sarah's larger than life personality, determination, courage, and resilience, she slowly began to come to terms with her condition and started to manage accept and pace, stating:

"A 5-minute walk is better than nothing, I need to try to channel this drive into a more positive effective energy which is not working against myself".

Through monitoring and exploring Sarah's thoughts, becoming aware of her own internal dialog and the impact this can have on her recovery. Her ability to be present and listening to her own body, showing self-compassion, practicing coping strategies (mindfulness, meditation, breathing) and building up trust in her abilities and confidence to manage, accept and pace has enabled Sarah to achieve what she expressed to me in 2011:

"I would like to write a book around M.E., my experience and possibly set up a support group".

As a therapist I feel engaging in therapy is probably one of the most difficult undertakings anyone can do, as we must look deep within ourselves and explore the difficult parts. I believe the client holds the elements to change within themselves and I provide the space, knowledge, and experience for the client to tap into their own world. The ability to take back control of their thoughts, feelings and responses has enabled Sarah to grow and achieve her goals.

Well done, Louise xx

One of the first things Louise got me to work on was acceptance. This was difficult work and there were a lot of tears, but in the end, I got there. The important thing is to grieve the losses and face the situation you are currently in. You never give up, but you adopt a better outlook that is freeing and less harmful to your body. You will notice that life gets a whole lot better. I stopped beating myself up over not being able to keep up with what I used to be able to do and took things at a more realistic pace. I looked on everything as an achievement and was grateful for any accomplishments I made.

Gratitude is an immensely powerful tool that I use daily as it makes everything so much better. Being grateful for the simple things like sounds, memories, textures, knowledge, smells, people etc. that you have in your life, is a wonderful feeling. It will result in you being much happier.

Louise and I worked through all the obstacles, one by one, and it helped enormously. I had to shrink everything down into manageable bites. After living a highly active life, the difficulty I had adjusting to my limitations got a little easier. The big things were:

- Being okay with just doing 5-minute walks on bad days.
- Admitting that I couldn't do something and having to ask for help.
- Saying NO to people.

My mindset now is to do what I can when I can. Anything else is destructive and will only mess with my body and mind. This condition limits us to a certain extent and needs readjustments to boundaries and lifestyle. It is important to remember to still do things at your own pace in your own way. Most of this book was written from my bed. Jim often found pens on his side of the bed when he lay down at night. I had heard of another person who had written a documentary from her bed. It is amazing what comes to mind when you set yourself free to explore the possibilities. I have been inspired by other people with this condition to try new things and I hope this book does the same for you.

Don't fight it! Just take responsibility and get on with life the best you can. The more you fight it the worse your situation will become, and you use up valuable energy.

Try some of the following:
• See the bigger picture. Step back and breathe. Have a look at things again.
• Try changing your outlook on life and enjoy each step. Introduce music etc.
• Be present, aware and focussed.
• Create space and breathe.
• Ask for advice and/or help from people you trust who have your best interest at heart.
• Build on what you are good at and what you love, and you won't go wrong.
Don't give up at the first sign of trouble. Keep going and work your way through it. You've got this.

OBSTACLES

BUILD CHARACTER AND
MAKE YOU STRONGER

As Louise and I worked through the process, I started to visualise setting up a self-help group near where I live. By doing this I worked out what it would involve. I then talked to Declan and together we managed to open it up in 2011 and it is still active. We are online now as times have changed due to Covid-19. We are all immune compromised, and it is not possible to meet in person as the risk is just too high at the moment due to Covid-19.

Being online via Zoom is fantastic as we can reach people all over the country.

START TODAY

You can decide today to get up and do something about your life that will benefit you. It doesn't have to be drastic. You can completely re-create yourself if you wish, one step at a time.

First, I had to come to terms with my condition and the effects it had on my life. I couldn't live the way I once did as my body wouldn't allow me to. I had to get my head around the challenges I faced and move on in a way that would allow me to come to terms with my limitations. When I was finishing up with Louise, we laughed at our final session as she told me that I was her most challenging client as serious adjustments had to be made. I had resisted at first but after good discussions, Louise helped me see how these changes would benefit me. It was difficult to adjust and calm down my free spirit. She compared me to a wild stallion who needed to be tamed. I finally got my head around certain areas, and the results were highly effective.

I am incredibly grateful for the help Louise gave me. My anger and frustration lessened enormously as I learnt different ways of thinking about things. I began to appreciate simple things like just being content going for a 5-minute walk, if that was all I was able for. Every effort is progress, as it takes lots of energy. Time management is paramount. I use my phone all the time now, setting the alarm so when doing any task, I allow myself a certain amount of time and then take a break. The results are I am not as exhausted, and my symptoms aren't as severe. Recurrences of immune system crashes have reduced also.
I began to say, "I want to do that, but can't do it all so let's find a way I can still do some of it". Take a simple thing like going out for the night with the girls. The whole night is out of the question for me as the payback would be horrendous. I began to meet up with them for two hours, resting earlier in the day and going straight to bed when I got home.

I love going to the beach. Normally I would have driven to the beach and walked the whole beach, which took about an hour to walk. I would then drive for an hour back home again. Now I get my husband to drive and I sleep on the way there and back and we walk for twenty minutes. Then we go for coffee before driving home again.

Everything can be maneuvered in this way. You just need to take it nice and easy and get lots of rest when you want to do something. You can pace at a rate that suits you. Nothing is permanent. Bad times don't last forever. You're not stuck. You have choices. Look at all the possibilities available to you. You can think new thoughts. You can learn something new if you wish. It might take a lot longer, but you will get there with patience and perseverance. Anything is possible if you put your mind to it. Be kinder to yourself. Learn how to take things at your own pace. Learn to take breathers, 5 minutes here and there to just be in the moment and clear your head. Introducing meditation is fantastic, just 2 minutes a day to start with. You can teach yourself new habits that will help you in the long run to be more content.

All that really matters is that you decide today to adjust your life for the better and then it will all fall into place. Once you start, you'll never need to stop.

I have learnt the journey has nothing to do with being nice, sure it is good to be nice, but it is about being real and authentic. Having boundaries is extremely important. Honour yourself and take care of your needs. In this mind frame being happy just happens and you do not fear what you can't control as much. I believe that once your heart is in the right place all else will flow.

Sit with your obstacles. Relax and let the answers come. Even though they are challenging and may make you feel like running, sit, give yourself time to breathe and take a good look at what solutions come to mind. You may not see a way through in the moment but sit with it and give it time. The answers will come.

MANAGING YOURSELF

BELIEVE YOU CAN! IF YOU'RE TIRED, REST, TOMORROW IS ANOTHER DAY! THE HOUSE WILL NOT FALL DOWN IF YOU DON'T UNLOAD THE DISHWASHER TILL TOMORROW. IT WILL STILL BE THERE, WAITING FOR YOU. GET A GOOD NIGHT'S SLEEP.

It is vital that we learn to take care of ourselves and balance out our lives. The results are we can care for others more effectively and be more content. Getting over tired from activities e.g. work, family, socialising etc. is going to lead to frustration and a short fuse which will be unpleasant for both you and the people around you.

Very few of us are in paid employment with this condition but if you are, take regular breaks. Get some fresh air as needed every couple of hours. In some countries there are sleep hubs at work, and it has proven very productive. The Spanish people take siestas. These are short naps taken in early afternoon after the midday meal. I am a big fan of siestas (one hour) and cat naps (fifteen minutes) when needed. For us, the one hour can lead to two. Sometimes I don't set an alarm, as I know I need as much sleep as I can get. I can sleep anything from 1 – 3 hours in the afternoon.

I would not recommend this if it interferes with your night's sleep. I can sleep this length and get a full nights uninterrupted sleep. Follow your own body and do what suits.

Work with your body. Listen to what it needs. Don't put yourself under too much pressure. Stress is not a good idea as it will exasperate your situation.

Self-awareness is your ability to accurately perceive your emotions and stay aware of them as they happen.

Self-management is your ability to use that awareness of your emotions to stay flexible and positively direct your behaviour.

It is not the trauma that defines us but how we choose to react to it. If we move on as opposed to remaining stuck, it will make a huge difference to our lives.

YOU CAN CREATE A PLACE OF PEACE AND SAFETY, NO MATTER WHERE YOU ARE.

With this condition, it is not always diagnosed quickly. You may feel you have it but don't yet have a diagnosis. If you are one of these people and you are reading this book, I hope you get sorted soon. Read through the following pages and pick what helps you.

A lot of people now may be at risk of getting M.E./CFS from Covid-19. Fatigue is a big issue with Covid-19. I have seen words like Covid-19 Longhaulers. These are people who after six to eight months are still experiencing extreme fatigue. The symptoms are quite similar to M.E./CFS. Things like cognitive problems with word finding, information processing, short term memory loss etc. These are all part of M.E./CFS. In the past many outbreaks of conditions like SARS and Ebola have resulted in the diagnosis of M.E./CFS.

Post infectious chronic illness is not a new thing. For those patients who may be developing M.E./CFS, please DO NOT try and push yourself or over-exercise/exert. This condition is drastically worsened by exertion of any kind. Listen to your body. Small activities like showering, dressing, housework, and computing can prove very difficult and if overdone will result in setbacks. I ended up in hospital with a huge migraine after trying to do a computer course in the early days. The teacher put pressure on me to do more as I could only do maximum of 20 minutes at a time. I pushed it to 45 minutes, and it backfired. This is called post-exertional malaise (PME) it is the main symptom of M.E./ CFS. This is where pacing comes in. Please see chapter on Pacing on page 70, for more information.

For those patients who may be developing M.E., you have probably noticed the 'midday slump'. That lack of energy you feel during the day. The feeling of being lethargic is not uncommon for us. You can improve that feeling. What we eat and when we eat is extremely important.

Here is what you can do for yourself to help feel more energetic:

1. Ask for help.
2. Eat healthy foods.
3. Get a good night's sleep.
4. Listen to your body.
5. Delegate.
6. Call a friend.
7. Space everything well out.
8. Eat light meals often.

Throughout this book there will be lots more suggestions on managing yourself.

I found finding a baseline a good start. This is where you feel at your best. Where you get things done and the level of pain and fatigue is at its lowest. It is not easy to keep at this level all the time but if you can stay within a range that suits you best as much as possible, life will be more pleasant. If you can look beyond your incapabilities and look at everything you have achieved so far in your life you will grow stronger. Your strength and your beautiful soul will shine for all to see.

NUTRITION

EATING WELL IS A FORM
OF SELF-RESPECT

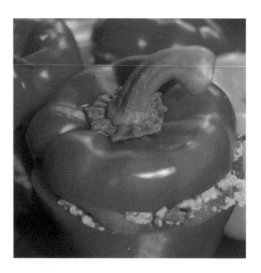

I have always been a good eater. When I started to look at food as medicine and how it can aid my body things started to change for the better.

It started back in 2013 when The Irish M.E. Trust had a therapy week in An Grianan ICA, in Co. Louth. A girl came to talk about how she had altered her eating pattern. The health benefits were fantastic.

I listened to how she changed to a clean diet where she removed toxic sprays and chemicals from her food and household products and ate organic fruit and vegetables etc. She got rid of all animal products, processed foods, and sweet sugary foods etc.

After I returned home I decided to make a few changes. I didn't want to switch too quickly as it would be overwhelming. I like to keep everything simple. My first goal was to eat vegetarian food 3 times a week. I also substituted some of my usual household products for environmentally friendly ones e.g. using vinegar and baking soda to clean. I found this was good, but after a few weeks I knew I had to go further as my health was not improving very much. After about a year I had reduced my meat and fish portions to once a week each. I had substituted my washing up liquid, weed killer, and deodorant. Most of my cleaning in the house was done with vinegar and baking soda.

By 2016 I realised I had to go further as my asthma was still awfully bad and I was on the maximum dose of medication. I had been to a specialist, but I was doing all I could do in her view.

Not long after, I was at home and my son, Sam, had returned from England, as the soccer season was on a break. I had just received a call about my cholesterol and it was not good. Sam had been listening in and asked me what was going on. He had also heard me coughing quite a lot since his return and was concerned. He suggested a plant-based diet. He had been changing over to this himself as it is used by lots of athletes to improve recovery and stamina and he felt it would be of benefit to me.

I hadn't a clue about this but liked the fact that giving up dairy apparently reduced phlegm in the body. If I could reduce the phlegm, then that would help me not to be choking so much when it built up.

We watched programmes on the benefits and did lots of research on it and I decided to give it a try. The most important thing with any changes to your eating pattern is to make sure you are getting the proper nutrition. I took a supplement every day of Vit B12. It wasn't that difficult to adjust over to a plant-based diet as alternatives are widely available and really tasty. I couldn't tell the difference to be honest between the dairy and dairy-free yogurt and ice-cream as they were delicious. I found the Linda McCartney's range of plant-based foods excellent.

After a while I noticed that there was a definite improvement in my body. The food was settling much better in my system and I didn't have that terrible bloated feeling. I had IBS for a long time and had got it under control, but my system had never worked so well as it was now. I knew there was no going back. The food was so tasty and the benefits to my body were so great that when I went for a body scan the results put a smile on my face for days. I had been watching Operation Transformation and the pharmacy near me called McCabes Pharmacy, were giving out free tests, so I decided to check it out. I was a bit nervous as I can't exercise too much with M.E./CFS. The most I do is a leisurely walk for about twenty minutes five days a week. I was thinking my body fat would be exceedingly high. I wasn't worried as I knew I could do something about that. As it happened things turned out very well. My actual age on the machine was 12 years younger than I was. This proved to me that food is everything. A little exercise and movement are important as well, of course, but get the food right and you're on the right track.

My asthma improved a lot. The build-up of phlegm that was causing havoc with my chest reduced. The choking lessened. I still have to use the inhalers, the nebuliser and all the medications when I get infections, but the big thing was that the phlegm had halved. I am so grateful that Sam was there that day and suggested switching as it has benefited me enormously.

There are lots of things you can eat, and you will find your energy along with your immune system will lift. Even if it's only slightly, it's progress and that's what we are after. You are moving in the right direction.

Anti-Inflammatory foods need to be a big part of your eating pattern. A classic sign of auto-immune conditions is inflammation in the body.

Foods like, broccoli, ginger, green leafy vegetables, blueberries, avocado, pineapple, and turmeric, help a lot. Just add a little of each to your meals throughout the week and you will notice a difference. The more you add the better the results.

I use turmeric a lot, it is fabulous for reducing inflammation. I take it in the evening before going to bed in some warm milk. I put half a spoon of turmeric powder, and a pinch of black pepper, in the bottom of a mug with a spoon or two of cold milk and stir till dissolved. I then add the heated milk into the mug with a bit of honey to sweeten. It helps a lot to fight the inflammation. The black pepper is especially important as it enhances the absorption of curcumin from the turmeric. This is a major advantage to your health.

Keep taking this as often as you can. You also get a great night's sleep which is an added bonus. You can add turmeric to most of your dishes e.g. curry, stews, slow cooker dishes, a tiny bit into your rice, or porridge, which gives a lovely colour.

Tips:
1. Eat naturally sweet foods like fruits.
2. Increase your vegetable intake.
3. Introduce a fist full of nuts and seeds daily.
4. Eat little and often.
5. Decrease red meat as it is hard for us to digest.

I am not saying cut meat out just cut back as it can be a lot of work for your body to digest and can cause that slump, I mentioned earlier. Try a couple of days a week on vegetarian / plant-based foods. Meat and dairy can be very heavy on the system. Don't worry, you won't be hungry.

Finally, increase your fibre. We all need more fibre in our meals. I use oat bran in my porridge and a spoonful in meals won't go astray.

Remember:
- Eat slowly
- Chew well
- Up your fibre
- Up your protein
- Down your sugar
- Reduce carbohydrates

- Increase herbs and spices.

The vitamins I choose to take the most are:

Vit C	Immunity/absorption of iron.
Vit B complex	Energy/Brain function/Cells metabolism/prevention of infections.
Vit D	Bones
Zinc	Absorption/immunity.
Magnesium	Regulates muscle and nerve function, blood sugar levels and blood pressure. Helps bones, energy, and ease muscle spasms.

In 1921, biochemist Casimir Funk was the first to use the term "vitamin" in a research publication that was accepted by the medical community.

"Sarah's Yumyums 101" on Facebook, Instagram, and YouTube has lots of quick easy nutritious dishes you may like.

DR. ROSAMUND VALLINGS

MHZM, MB BS (LOND), MRCS LRCP,
DIP CLIN HYP, BA (MASSEY).

Dr. Rosamund Vallings is one of the leading authorities on Chronic Fatigue Syndrome (M.E./CFS) in New Zealand. I have had the pleasure of meeting Ros on several occasions when she visited Ireland. She has given many talks for the Irish ME Association over the years. I hope to see her again as she is a lovely lady.

Ros has kindly allowed me to share with you her top five tips for helping us manage M.E./CFS:

1. *If you have symptoms of postural orthostatic tachycardia syndrome POTS (orthostatic intolerance) such as dizziness on standing in the heat, getting up suddenly or tendency to feel faint, make sure you have plenty of salt. This should be through the day – say a helping or pinch of salt every 2 -3 hours. Drink adequately but not too much as that can wash the salt and other electrolytes out. Get your blood pressure checked regularly. If you already have high blood pressure the extra salt is not for you.*
2. *A snack at bedtime can help improve quality of sleep in M.E./CFS according to sleep researcher Martin Partinen. This helps the orexin system – a brain system which is related to sleep quality. Most people with M.E./ CFS do not have quality sleep, and usually wake feeling unrefreshed even*

if they have slept many hours. Magnesium at bedtime can be an added help too – sleep is more restful, and symptoms such as crampy pain are often alleviated. Take about 300mg.

3. Low dose Naltrexone seems a worthwhile drug to try, as long as it blends with other drugs you need to take. They have found it quietens down the inflammation in the brain and has some benefit to correcting the immune system abnormalities discovered by the team at Griffith University in Queensland, Australia.

4. It is vital that you do not over-exercise. There is a great temptation to do more if you start to feel better. But you can easily push it too hard too soon. So do pace yourself very carefully. So many people learn the hard way and relapse by trying to do too much and progress too rapidly. So always test yourself out very carefully. The supplement Coenzyme Q10 has been shown to enhance the muscle mitochondria and help to relieve muscle pain and weakness. But it is not for everyone and can be quite expensive. About 200mg should be taken in the morning.

5. Stress management should always be included in your recovery plan. This does not mean that the illness is all due to stress but handling stress will give you a better chance of maintaining improvement and avoiding relapse. It is something we all need to focus on for life! Some form of daily relaxation is always worthwhile. There are many suitable options to consider – Try out lots of possibilities and find out which suits you – Then practice daily. Ideas would include, meditation, mindfulness, self-hypnosis, yoga (not too strenuous). The Limerick group have tried Therapeutic Yoga and found it excellent. Again, do it at your own pace. More ideas include, Tai Chi, deep abdominal breathing while listening to music, playing a musical instrument and stroking an animal – the stroking action induces endorphin release for the animal (e.g. cats purr) and the hand stroking give you stimulation effects to produce endorphins for you too.

BOUNDARIES

IF SOMEONE THROWS A FIT BECAUSE YOU SET BOUNDARIES, IT'S JUST MORE EVIDENCE THAT BOUNDARIES ARE NEEDED.

When I think of boundaries, I see in my mind the giant aqua bubble that you step into that allows you to roll on water. No one can get near you, but they can bounce off your bubble. The important thing is to know you are in charge of who and what comes into your bubble.

It is particularly important to set boundaries for yourself. If you are in a situation and you notice someone's mood change and you begin to feel uncomfortable, this is the time to either find an excuse or, move on from the situation.

A simple, "Can you excuse me?" or "I need to go to the bathroom", or "Can we agree to differ on that?" and move on. You can pick whatever you wish and use it at the appropriate time. The aim is to not be in a stressful situation that makes you feel uncomfortable.

Once you let people know what you don't accept, e.g. it's not okay to speak to me that way, then it's up to you to call them out on the behaviour when it arises. You may also need to tell them the consequences for breaking those boundaries, e.g. if they continue with this behaviour you will walk away.

When dealing with Boundaries you will need to learn to say NO! to yours and others bad behaviour.

A lot of people aren't aware of this condition which results in lack of understanding and compassion. How we handle this is important.

If you are trying to have a conversation with someone about something you do not like - be clear in your communication. If they start insulting you, say "Stop, no insulting allowed". If they start cursing at you or the tone changes you may need to say, "let's get back to the point" You must stay calm. You might need to leave it for another day if they are not willing to be respectful towards you. There is no point in getting into an argument. If you don't tolerate it from a child don't tolerate it from an adult.

You need to define your boundaries, and this means sitting down and writing them out, so you are clear with yourself what you will tolerate. If you are clear with yourself, it will be easier to be clear with others.

Sometimes you will be emotional about things. For me it is the harming of children and animals. Other times it will be the way people treat you. There must be a line in the sand and if they cross it, you need to protect yourself.

Another way of looking at boundaries is like a game of tennis. You are on one side of the net and the person who is challenging your boundaries is on the other side. The net is your guideline. You decide how close to the net you go before you stop acting in a way that is infringing on your personal boundaries of self-care. For example, how far you will go before you overdo things and get exhausted. The net for your tennis partner is how far you will let them go before they reach the net. Most of us have someone in our life, that is continuously trying to wind us up or just plain nasty, rude, or bulling towards you. It could also be a friend who is not clear on your physical boundaries. Make it clear to them what behaviour is acceptable and what isn't so they don't get too near the net. If they still cross the line, remind them of the consequences of these actions. It's important to follow through. For example, you visit your neighbour, and every time they are grumpy and disrespectful towards you. Inform them that if they want you to visit as regularly as you have been, they need to be more pleasant and if they start to be unpleasant you will have to leave. Chances are they don't even realise they are doing it but after a couple of times of you leaving early, they'll get the message.

It takes courage but it can be done as you must protect yourself and you deserve to be respected. Boundaries are an act of self-care.

Be confident in your ability to deliver these boundaries. Confidence can go up and down based on your emotions, hence the name "wave of emotion". Stay clear and focus on what you want to say, and you will be fine. Be aware of your emotions and work on not letting them go to high or too low. Adjust them as needed. Breathe. Once you're calm, you'll find things a lot easier to manage. Please note that all communication must be carried out in a calm and respectful manner as fighting is not going to help you or your energy.

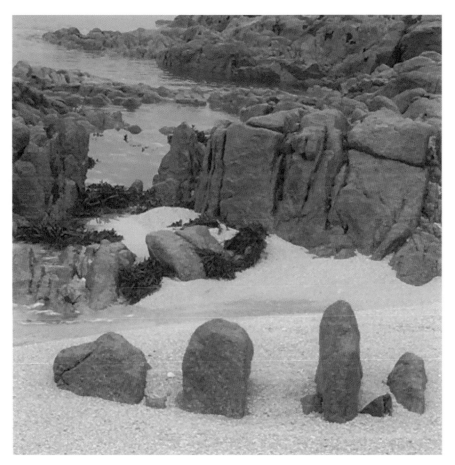

PACING

EVERY FLOWER BLOOMS IN ITS OWN TIME AND AT ITS OWN PACE

Once I came to terms with managing my M.E./CFS I started to pace myself better and noticed little improvements. I knew then that I was on the right track. The frequency of the flare ups started to reduce. Instead of dips every week and flare-ups every few months I noticed I was getting away with a bit more. Flareups now happened every few months. It all depended on how much I did. I had to find my level that worked for me and caused the least amount of pain, nausea, and extreme fatigue. I cut back on a lot of things. Just doing what I needed to do and not push myself too much. I listened to what my body was telling me. This helped a lot.

Pacing is about learning what level of activity suits your particular body. Everyone will differ. Find a level that gives you the best balance, so you don't become floored as regularly.

The key is to stop before you become over tired. I get heaviness/dull pain between my eyes, stiffness in the back of my neck and slowness in my speech. I mix up words and I am not able to think straight. When this starts to happen, it's time to stop what I'm doing and sit, rest or get some sleep. It all depends on the level of fatigue I am experiencing.

When someone asks me, "What is M.E./CFS like?" or "How do I

pace myself?" I use 2 comparisons:

1. Battery: M.E./CFS is like having a half charged battery all the time that runs down very fast and needs to be charged up regularly (rest/pacing yourself) You can also conserve your energy while awake e.g. talk less, listen more' delegate and ask for help.

2. Bank: Anytime you spend money (energy) you must pay it back (rest / pacing yourself)

PACING YOURSELF IS VITAL. SET AN ALARM IF YOU MUST.

When practicing pacing yourself, you can get more done once you find a level/balance that works for you.

I dislike tidying out cupboards a lot! For me to do it, I set aside twenty minutes a day until the task is done. First, I set an alarm for twenty minutes. I stop when the alarm goes off. That way I don't feel overpowered and overfatigued. If I overdo it, it leads to frustration anger and pain and I don't touch the task again for days and sometimes longer. This does not happen when I pace myself and I actually get more done.

Make a list of what you want to do and do the most important things first. I try to do my tasks first thing in the morning as that is my best time of the day. You can choose yours. When you have your task done you can tick it off your to do list. This is a great feeling.

Some days when you feel physically and emotionally low and unable to face the tasks you need to do, that's okay. Take it nice and easy that day and you will be able to face the tasks tomorrow or the next day. Just don't get into the habit of putting things off too much, as that leads you into procrastination which is another area which we will be talking about in the next chapter.

I have found that the best thing for getting tasks completed is to start small.

Plan your day. Give yourself 2 minutes the night before. I usually make a note in the calendar in my phone. Allow yourself different times for tasks e.g.

Clearing out cupboards – 10 mins

Work on project - 15 mins
Clean hot press – 10 mins
Exercise – 10 mins or less, (everything is an achievement)
Reading a new book – 5 mins
If there is something you must get done but don't feel like doing, do 1 min to start.

You will find once you start small you will go back to it and before you know it, you will have achieved lots. You will be delighted with yourself.

When I started writing this book I did so for fifteen minutes a day. Sometimes I missed a day, but I came back when I was able. With this condition we get regular times when we are not able to do a lot. You will find when you pace yourself, nice and slow, it helps a lot. Pain cuts down, that bone crushing fatigue hits less often as you learn to stop before you overdo it. The less you do the better. I realise we all have things to do but if you live in a house with other family members, delegate and ask for help.

MANAGE YOUR DAY BY DIVIDING IT INTO SECTIONS:
PACING YOURSELF IS YOUR PRIORITY, ALWAYS!

Here is an example of my pacing:
• Rise at 8am (You can do 10 minutes of visualisation before you get out of bed.)
• 9am Breakfast
• 10am Walk, whatever distance you are able for, you decide. 5 – 10 minutes is good daily. Even indoor exercise helps.
• 11am Tea/Coffee break. Sit outside if you can. Day light is very therapeutic.
• 11.30am Clean Kitchen. Pace yourself e.g. twenty minutes
• 12am Reading. Start with five minutes daily.
• 1pm Lunch + fifteen minutes cat nap
• 2pm Meet a friend
• 3.30pm Rest (with ten minutes of meditation before you sleep)

- 5pm get dinner ready
- 7pm Watch TV
- 8pm Have bath and then bed

Now, like I said this is only a sample and it will differ for everyone daily. Do what you're able for and the plan of your day is up to you. Having some structure is important. My specialist Dr. Mary Ryan recommended that it is good to get up at the same time each day and go to bed 12 hours later. So, if you're up at 9am go to bed at 9pm. This will take some time to adjust to so work on it slowly. You can go for naps in between. Some days I get up, dressed, and eat breakfast only to turn around and go back to bed as I'm just not feeling well at all, and that's fine. Listen to your body and give yourself permission to do what is best for you.

The golden rule of pacing is:
Whatever you think you can do, halve it, and halve it again. Make that your starting point.

WALK THROUGH LIFE. DON'T WORRY ABOUT WHAT OTHERS ARE DOING. DO IT AT YOUR OWN PACE. IT'S YOUR BODY SO LISTEN TO IT, THEN ACT.

SELF-BELIEF

"YOU CAN ALWAYS FIND SOMETHING TO BE HAPPY
ABOUT EVERY DAY, EVEN IF ONLY FOR A FEW MINUTES.
LOOK ON THE BRIGHT SIDE OF THINGS AND
HAVE A LAUGH WHENEVER POSSIBLE"

Helping each other to have the confidence and self belief

In the beginning of 2011, I realised I needed to start doing something to help others with this condition. My confidence had risen, and I believed I could help others do the same.

I figured that if I did something 2 hours a week that would be a start. So, with the backing of The Irish M.E. Trust we opened Limerick's first support group for people with M.E./CFS. I called it Limerick ME self-help support group. We met once a week. The aim was to help people feel better. They now had somewhere to go where they could get advice on how to improve their quality of life. Different speakers came and gave wonderful advice which proved extremely helpful.

Loneliness and depression are part of this condition as our lives have been altered dramatically. Having people gather that understood what we were going through was a great help to us all. One thing I wanted to make sure of was that people left the group feeling better than when they arrived. Thankfully, that was the case. Sure, we talked about the difficult things we experienced, the challenges we faced but we always found room for laughter, gratitude, and appreciation for what we did have and what we could do. The great thing is we learnt from each other and were there for each other as well. There was always something we could do to improve our quality of life.

Surround yourself with people that lift you up

The right people will give you confidence and strong self-belief. Be careful with the people you surround yourself with. If people are bothering you, don't be afraid to walk away if you need to, as it is very powerful, and sends a clear message. You will find as time goes by, they won't bother you as much. This results in you having better relationships in your life. The ones you choose. Your past is another thing you must not be afraid to leave behind.

You may need to walk away from all the drama and people who create it. Surround yourself with people who make you laugh. Forget the bad and focus on the good. Love the people who treat you right. Increase the time you spend with them as this will give you joy. Hang around with those who lift you up not those who bring you down.

My rule is:

If they lift you up, keep them but if they bring you down, limit your time with them. Life is just too short, and we must enjoy our time and not waste it unnecessarily. Take a deep breath in and believe that you can do anything you put your mind to and say

"I CAN DO THIS"

Your internal vocabulary is especially important. If this is negative, you're never going to get far. It is easy to work on, just be aware of your thoughts and don't worry if at first you find it's not great. The more time you work on this the better it gets. Start today. Remember it takes a while to form a new habit. Don't be too hard on yourself as you are a work in progress.

You can do this!

Self-belief is particularly important. We've all heard the stories, the miracles e.g. the person who's told after an accident they will never walk again, and they do! It's not always true what you are told by the specialist as there are people who have beaten the odds before and walked again. It happens and no one can explain it.

Be crystal clear in your beliefs and wishes. Decide what you want in specific detail and go for it with complete self-belief. Step by step, take it slow. Be mindful of your limitations and pace yourself. Keep dreaming and visualising what you want. Our imagination is unlimited.

I dreamed about going back skiing for years but now I visualise about going on a ski mobile. I had to tweak that one a little as it wasn't happening, but I replaced it with another dream and that is important as you have to dream about doing things. It cheers you up.

I can't emphasise enough the importance of pacing as this condition is unforgiving. If you pace, your body will thank you and you will have less setbacks. You will find the level that suits you regarding what you can do. I know how frustrating this can be. If you tweak your thoughts and be grateful for what you can do, this will benefit you. In doing so, you will reduce, stress, anxiety, and frustration. We need to face our reality we are in. That way we can open ourselves to the new things that are coming into our lives.

Acknowledge what it is, and then do what you can to improve your life. Have your dreams. See what you want. Feel it, visualise it, and don't let negativity put you off. Never give up!

I dream of getting better. I focus on what I want e.g. being able to do the things everyone takes for granted, like going to work, going on long walks without paying a price for it. No nausea, no dizziness. In my dreams I get up at 8am and go to bed at 9pm, not having to watch or pace everything in between. There are no limits as it's my imagination and I can go anywhere and do anything I wish. I accept life as it is now, but I will never give up on the dream.

Enjoy the trips you take in your mind as they send good vibes to your body. I do believe that the day will come, hopefully soon, where I will not be so limited in my activities. There is a lot more focus on M.E./CFS these days and that gives me hope.

We always have to believe it will come and, in the meantime, we will do what is best for us, so our bodies are in good shape and our minds are strong.

REST, RECOVERY, AND REFLECTION
ARE ESSENTIAL PARTS OF THE PROGRESS TOWARDS
A HAPPY LIFE.

Feeling comfortable within yourself is a game changer.

Do you ever feel like you're doing the same thing day in and day out? That's because your mind wants what is familiar, so it feels safe. The thing is we come across unfamiliar things every day and that forces us to do one of two things, retreat or go for it.

For example, feeling uncomfortable when receiving a compliment. Do you feel uncomfortable when you are complimented by other people?

If you are not used to getting compliments and it feels strange, this is something you can turn around. We can do one of two things. Enjoy it or shy away from it and say something to put yourself down e.g. "this old thing, I got this for half 'nothing'.

Can you hear yourself?

I used to be like this until I changed things up and started receiving compliments with gratitude. It is lovely to get compliments, we can enjoy them too. The intention of the person giving you the compliment is to make you feel good inside. Try it and see for yourself. I started by just saying "Thank You" and feeling the lovely feeling of getting the compliment and do you know what? I kept doing that, and now I love when people compliment me, and I feel great. No more uncomfortable feelings, just nice warm feelings. I often ask myself : "Why didn't I do this earlier?"

Wear what makes you feel good and walk tall and smile, because if you believe you are fabulous then others will see it as well and say it.

Here are a few suggestions:

GIVE YOURSELF A COMPLIMENT every morning while brushing your teeth. It may feel uncomfortable, but it is very necessary. Things like:

"I am beautiful inside and out"

"I can do a good job"

"I am strong enough"

"I am a kind, loving, and likable person"

"I am a very capable person" etc.

This might feel unnatural at first but stick with it as you will adjust, and your confidence will lift and that is what you are after. Try and do it for 30 days to start.

Stack your habits

This is where we build habits in twos or threes. e.g.

• Wash your hands and name three things you are grateful for and stretch when finished.

• Cook dinner and listen to Podcasts.

• Put on your moisturiser and state your intention for the day ahead.

Banish self criticism

We are ridiculously hard on ourselves and this makes us miserable and that in turn make us unpleasant to others around us. When you notice yourself being unkind to yourself and saying things like.

• "I'm too…"

• "I don't like my…",

• "I hate the way I…"

STOP! You have the power to change your beliefs.

Write down:

3 positive beliefs you have and 3 negative ones. Work on the negative ones, flip them, and be constantly aware of future behaviour so you can continuously change your unwanted patterns. You can use the three positive beliefs to manage the three negative ones.

_____

_____

_____

_____

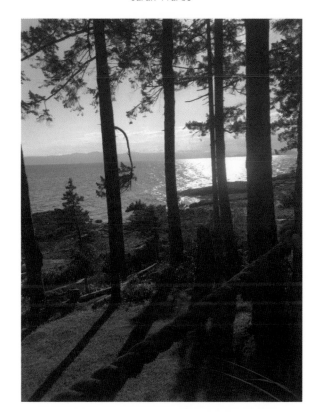

ENJOY THE PACE OF NATURE

Here are some examples where you can help yourself to feel better:
- Start believing that you can do anything you put your mind to.
- Love yourself for who you are.
- If you are unhappy about your weight e.g. you wish to lose 2 stone, you can visualise yourself at your ideal weight and tell yourself that you are that weight. Your brain doesn't know the difference. You have a better chance of getting to the desired weight if you do this. Then make a conscious decision to choose the right foods.
- It's all about the choices you make. The same goes for everything you do.
- If you choose to look and think about things in a better light, the way you feel will shift and improve.
- Choose uplifting and supportive language like:

I will …………..
I can ……
I am intelligent
I am good enough and always will be

THERE ARE MANY WINDOWS IN A MANSION, EACH ONE
GIVES A DIFFERENT VIEW AND ANGLE OF WHAT LIES
BEYOND. CHOOSE TO LOOK OUT THE WINDOW THAT
GIVES THE BEST VIEW FOR YOU.

GRATITUDE

I love Oprah. I listen to her a lot. She has had an incredibly positive and uplifting effect on my life. Between listening to Oprah and Tony Robbins I believe that this is one of the reasons I am so strong and able to deal with life and its challenges. I learnt how to be more grateful by watching Oprah. I decided to up the ante on this a few years ago and see what effect it would have. I am happy to say the results were incredibly positive. Gratitude now plays a big role in all my life.

I started off by saying things like:
1. Thank you for the car I drive. It's so much better for me than getting the bus
2. Thank you for the food I eat every day
3. Thank you for the roof over my head
4. Thank you for the wonderful people in my life
5. Thank you for being alive

And on and on and on it goes. In the past I wouldn't remember every day to be grateful but a couple of times a week I'd practice it. I started by writing down what I was grateful for.

A few years ago, my son bought me a Gratitude Journal and that was a turning point. Every night before I went to sleep, I would write down at least 3 things I was grateful for that day. My sleep improved threefold as my mind was full of good things.

Now, when going through the day and something good happens I say a quick thank you to the universe and move on. It's become a habit that has improved my quality of life as I am much more content.

We can take a lot of things for granted. We may complain about being stuck in traffic, being bored, waiting in queues in shops, etc. These are little things that we can get upset about when there is no need. What good does it do you? Getting upset isn't going to serve you. If anything, it's going to make you worse off. Take a moment to breathe and refocus and ask yourself: "What do I need to do now?"

Then, make a decision. You can accept and move on in a calmer manner when you have decided what to do. This does take time to master but it will become easier as you develop the habit.

I tell my husband not to sweat the small stuff as it is a complete waste of time and energy. We need to be careful not to waste our energy.

Anger is a secondary emotion. Ask yourself what is feeding the anger? I was told before to see anger as a rock. Turn it over and look underneath and see what lies beneath. Is it frustration, hurt, fear, guilt, feeling powerless? These all make you feel anger. You need to investigate which one is the cause. The anger covers up the feelings so you must take time and figure it out so that you can understand. Once you know the cause you can work on the solution. Maybe you are blaming yourself for something or you are fearful of a certain outcome. Find out what is bothering you and you will feel so much better. There is an answer to everything and a way around each situation. It may just need a little time and a pen and paper. Let all your thoughts out. Set them free.

In times of frustration and anger, try finding something to be grateful for. It is amazing how it turns the situation around. There is always something to be grateful for.

PEOPLE HAVE OPINIONS
NO MATTER WHAT YOU DO. LET THEM.
DO WHATEVER BRINGS YOU JOY
AND LIVE YOUR LIFE ON YOUR TERMS.

STEPS TO TAKE TO HELP YOURSELF:

1 Be aware
2 Accept the situation you are in
3 Articulate what you want
4 Make a plan
5 Take action and watch things change
6 Be grateful that you achieved your results

Gratitude is a positive state leading to better health so the more we appreciate the things that are around us the better our quality of life can be. Be aware of how you feel when you are grateful. Take note of things you are grateful for daily. It is an enormously powerful exercise, and it puts your mind in a wonderful state. If you can form this habit it can benefit you enormously.

Appreciation
Complaining about our situation won't get us anywhere. It will waste a lot of energy and makes us feel worse. Instead of complaining try and look at what is working in your life right now. We can realise how lucky we are and figure out a way to solve what we are complaining about and move on. We need to realise what we can control and let the rest go. We can have a tendency to complain about things that have nothing to do with us. Start taking action and responsibility for your own things and leave other people to sort out theirs.

How do you treat your best friend? You do right by them, and are kind and loving towards them, right? Well that's how you need to treat yourself. We must do what we think is the right thing, otherwise we harm ourselves and others. What I do during my day sends signals back to me about what kind of person I am.

You can't get away from it. If you do things that are wrong, you will think about it and therein lies the problem. You pay when you don't do what you think is the right thing. Start to pay attention to the vibes and feelings that you're getting on a daily basis. They tell you a lot.

ALWAYS REMEMBER PEOPLE WILL LOVE YOU
PEOPLE WILL HATE YOU AND NONE OF IT WILL HAVE
ANYTHING TO DO WITH YOU. YOU CAN'T PLEASE EVERY-
ONE SO JUST DO WHAT YOU FEEL IS GOOD FOR YOU
AND TAKE CARE OF YOURSELF THEN YOU CAN TAKE
BETTER CARE OF OTHERS.

EXPRESS YOURSELF

HAVE THE CONFIDENCE
TO FREE YOURSELF
TO BE 100% YOU!

Get it out!

It is particularly important to express yourself. Bottling things up can be unbelievably bad for you. I used to let things slide, so as not to rock the boat. All I wanted was peace and quiet but the problem with that was that things would build up and I would get terribly angry. This left me exhausted.

One day my husband sat me down and told me to let him know when I was not happy with something when it occurred, not to keep it inside and let it build up, as it was not good for either of us. I must say he was right. Now I don't bottle things up. If I am not happy with something I simply say, "Just letting you know I'm not happy with…" That way he knows, and we can discuss things and come to an understanding we are both happy with. It works so much better and I'm not wasting energy. Communication is key.

Expectation leads to disappointment. If you want something, say it. Don't presume as people can't read your mind. You might not always get what you want but at least you verbalised it and that's a lot better than keeping it in and sending bad harmful vibes through your body and mind. This helps to prevent anger, frustration and disappointment.

There will be painful moments in your life that will change your entire world in a matter of minutes. Let them make you stronger, smarter, and kinder. You don't want to become someone who is bitter, resentful, and angry all the time. Cry, scream, do what you must but let it go and learn from it. Then straighten up and get on with life with your head held high because you are still here, so make the most of the hand you are dealt. Keep moving forward and be grateful for the lesson life gives you. You have survived this far. You've got this.

Be brave:

Don't let others disrespect you. If they do, find a way to express how you feel. Try saying "I love you, but it hurts me when you..." Or "I felt hurt by the way you..." The most important thing is to get it out and don't bottle it up. You just end up revisiting the conversation repeatedly in your head for days. You hear yourself saying "Why didn't I say ...".

Try this:

Imagine that the person is in the room with you, right in front of you. Talk to them and say what you want to say. You need to really get into this and feel it. This is a great exercise because when you eventually meet them to say what it is you need to say, it will come out much more relaxed. If it is the case that you can't face them as they are too confrontational that's ok. This exercise can get your thoughts out and you expressing yourself.

You can also say that this behaviour shows you that they are unhappy and ask them what happened to make them so. I learnt this from my mother. There was a nun in a hospital that everyone was afraid of. She worked in reception and you had to pass her to get into visit people. One day my mum asked her was she ok, had something happened to upset her. The nun looked shocked and there was silence. My mum stayed quiet and the nun eventually spoke. When she did, she expressed that yes, she was very unhappy and did not enjoy the work she was doing and wished she could move to a different section. My mum chatted away to her for a while and they arranged to meet again to see what may be done to help her. The nun eventually moved to a new position and was much more content and they remained friends.

The reason I tell this story is because you just don't know what is going on in others' lives and secondly if you are not happy in a situation you can change it.

FOCUS

THIS CONDITION CAN TEST US, IT WILL KNOCK US DOWN BUT WE ARE STRONG ENOUGH TO GET UP AND FACE LIFE AGAIN TOMORROW.

Focus on what you can do to help yourself. Look at how you want to feel and what you will do to improve your quality of life and your state of mind. Stay on track and keep moving forward with what you want.

This will help you:
When a negative thought enters your mind, once you become aware of it, think of three positive ones. This will counteract the negativity. Train yourself to flip the script. This will improve how you feel instantly.

Staying focussed on what you want to do is important. Therefore, have a to do list.
I usually have 3 things a day that I prioritise on my list. I don't want to get overfatigued, so I keep it short. The list is great to keep me focussed and when I have completed the tasks on my list, I feel a lovely sense of achievement.
Get moving. This is an achievement. Even if it's as small as getting up to move every hour. Walk around the house. Sitting for long peri-

ods is awfully bad for you.

Days can slip away from me if I don't focus on what it is, I wish to get done. I find I spend less time on less important things and don't get distracted as much. With lists, it reminds me what needs to be done. I have learnt not to beat myself up too much if I do not get all the tasks done as I can move them to the next day. A smile comes on my face each time I tick off an item on the list.

Ask yourself, "What do I need to get done right now?" Even with all the planning, things can happen that are beyond our control. Life just comes in and takes over and that is okay. If you want to do something just do it and take the plunge as it will be what it will be. You can figure it out along the way. Have a goal and a plan and the rest is all about action. Flexibility is important.

Set reminders on your phone or on sticky notes. For example, write down:

Your top 3 most important tasks to be completed today.

Your goals for the week, well spread out.

Who you would like to call or visit this week?

Tell a friend:

This will help make it real and motivate you into completing what needs to be done. I found it difficult to stick to anything for a long period of time. Usually at about 4 to 6 weeks I lost interest. I started using these techniques a few years ago and they helped me enormously. I am not saying I am completely flawless, far from it; but they keep me on track most of the time. It is important to be encouraged along the way.

Find someone you are close to; a friend you can call any time or a family member. If you are e.g. trying to eat healthy, you can encourage and motivate each other. This can really help. Chat daily and give each other tips on how to get through the day.

Keep an eye on the time. Don't let it run away with you. If you get overtired, it is difficult to do anything for a couple of days. It is important to walk away from a task after the allotted time, say fifteen minutes, and come back to it the following day if you feel up to it. Don't let yourself get over tired.

These tasks can be whatever you want. Here are a few examples: When cleaning the house, go room by room. Plan your week. Don't try to do it all at once as this will aggravate your fatigue. Do one room a day.

IT DOESN'T MATTER HOW SLOWLY YOU GO AS LONG
AS YOU GET TO WHERE YOU WANT TO GO.

When you are clearing out paperwork, set a timer for twenty minutes a day. That is a lot of time over a week but remember, if you do it all at once you may get over tired.

It is important that you enjoy what you are doing and make your environment as pleasant as possible. Make sure you are cool/warm enough. Put on some music. Be aware of yourself and your surroundings while you do whatever it is you are doing.

Do your task and then do something nice like:
- Get some fresh air for 5 minutes.
- Have a cup of tea.
- Listen to the birds sing.
- Dance.
- Breathe and be grateful for what you have achieved.

If you are fully focussed on the task at hand, you will find you will get a lot done and enjoy it. In time you will find you can do a little bit more and your concentration will grow. Remember you can adjust the times to suit yourself. A maximum of twenty minutes is enough no matter how well you feel. You want to continue with it the following day so easy does it. If you are getting the job done, that's what is important. So, step by step. You will win the race in the end. You are in control of the situation. Now, doesn't that feel good?

THE BEST THINGS IN LIFE ARE THE PEOPLE YOU LOVE,
THE PLACES YOU'VE SEEN AND THE MEMORIES
YOU'VE MADE ALONG THE WAY

Talk to people who believe in you and leave all the others go. You need to be encouraged, not put down or put off. People can be full of negativity and that's not going to do you any good at all. If you have a dream, no matter how small, go for it and don't let anyone's opinion put you off.

Keep the dream alive.

I find motivation clips on YouTube help me a lot. I also read and listen to Ted Talks on the subjects that interest me. I love to listen to music and watch movies that lift me up, especially if I am down in the dumps. Try watching TV when ironing, and, listening to music while food shopping.

Help somebody and be kind. Doing good does you good. Have fun and reward yourself for getting the job done. If there is something particular you want to get done, adjust the time you are spending on e.g. TV, Facebook, Laptop, etc. Replace what you want to do e.g. writing, reading, drawing, meditation, art, etc. You decide.

EMBRACE THE WONDERFUL PERSON YOU ARE

Remember:
- You've got this.
- The "I Can Do it" attitude will get you far.
- Be patient.
- Positive grounded thinking helps.
- Moaning and groaning doesn't help.
  We all know what our ailments are, we don't need to focus on them.
- Focus on what will benefit you.
- Learn how to tackle issues in a manner that will benefit you.
- Flip your mood.
- You have unique qualities, take a good look at yourself.
- You have greatness inside that fear is stopping. Find the greatness.
- Speak more kindly to yourself & others.
- Laugh out loud.
- Open your heart.
- Smile brightly.

- Breathe deeply.
- Listen.
- Hug tightly.
- Stop being so uptight and serious.
- Take your time. There is no rush.
- Stop making excuses.
- Stop being a victim. Stand strong.
- Stop letting people bring you down.
- Make a decision to protect yourself.
- If anyone puts pressure on you tell them to stop.

Be enthusiastic about life. Every day is a fresh start, a new beginning, a gift. No looking back, as that is in the past, it's gone. You will find this extremely exciting. It will give a clean sheet daily.

You have the freedom to choose. So many opportunities will come your way and you can choose to take them. You have the choice each day to pick what's best. You can stay in the situation you're in or plan a different route. Anything is possible if you put your mind to it. There is always room for improvement. You can have a better quality of life by making the appropriate changes. Small steps in the right direction can make the world of difference. You can mend the wounds of the past bit by bit until they heal. Make life easier on yourself, by being kind and understanding, to yourself and others. Have fun looking at the endless possibilities that are in front of you and pick what suits you.

Start today:

Smiling is infectious. Give someone the gift of a smile today! When someone smiles at you, you can't help smiling back. When you think of smiling, it puts a smile on your face and before you know it you feel better. A single smile can travel around faster than you could ever think. If you feel a smile coming, bring it on, share it and watch it travel. See how many smiles you can pass on to others. This will make you smile even more. Here is a poem I found that is beautiful.

Sarah Warde

Infectious Smiles:

Smiling is infectious
You catch it like a flu
When someone smiled at me today
I started smiling too
I walked around the corner
And someone saw me grin
When he smiled I realised
I had passed it on to him
I thought about the smile
And then realised its worth
A single smile like mine
Could travel round the earth
So, if you feel a smile begin
Don't leave it undetected
Start an epidemic
And get the world infected
Jez Alborough

FIND OUT WHAT BUILDS YOUR ENTHUSIASM
AND MAKE A LIST.

SELF-CARE

DON'T WAIT TO CHANGE
START NOW!

Self-Care is extremely important always. We need to work on it continuously. Not just our personal things like our hair, clothes grooming, but our inner self-care. The inner voice that chatters all day in your ear. I call it my angel and devil.

As kids we were told how to focus on one and the other would die down. Be kind and patient with yourself. This can be challenging at times but if you can just work on it and come from a loving place, things can be easier.

Control the controllables.

There are only some things within our control. The rest we can do nothing about. So be aware of what you have control over and what you don't have control over and chuck the rest in "the fuck it bucket" This can be very freeing. Try it.

We all need love and understanding. Be gentle with yourself. Focussing on self-care is vital. If you don't look after yourself, how do you expect to look after the people around you effectively?
An important part of self-care is how we manage criticism.

Let's look at the 3 types of criticism:

1. Self-criticism
2. Destructive criticism
3. Constructive criticism

Learning how to deal with each and understanding them is particularly important if we are going to look after ourselves properly.

Self-criticism

Self-criticism is by far the worst! Self-criticism is the voice in your head that says "you can't do this" or "you're not good enough" or "they don't like you" etc.

You need to change that inner voice. Change it to someone who loves you no matter what.

Choose a supportive understanding voice inside your head. One who has got your back. Love yourself. Your inside voice can be your biggest critic or your best friend.

Reassure yourself by saying things like:
- Go for it!
- I can do this!
- I've got this!
- I am good enough!

My favourite affirmation is from a girl I went to school with, Rosemary. She always told herself, "You're as good as many and better than most!" I still use this.

Flip the script from negative to positive. Instead of saying "I've a terrible memory" you say, "I've a great memory"

WHAT YOU TALK ABOUT YOU BRING ABOUT.

Negative / destructive criticism

Many of us have people in our lives who criticise us regularly. We need to learn to not let that in. This can be challenging but we can succeed. Criticism that comes from another shows you how miserable that person is. They may constantly criticise themselves, setting unrealistic standards and finding fault with everything. They are very unhappy.

When they criticise you, flip it over and thank them. Recognise the criticism for what it is. Let it fall onto an imaginary tray that you are holding in the palm of your hand. Hand the invalid criticism back by saying the opposite for example, someone says "you're lazy" the response is "no, I'm not lazy, in fact I'm extremely hard working".

Don't get defensive. Don't fall into the trap. Stand up tall and express yourself in a calm assertive manner.

Constructive criticism

Focus on the positive part of the criticism and plan to work on the rest.

Constructive criticism is good and if it is valid it will help you to develop and grow. Look on it as advice e.g. "I love the way you wrote that; would it be clearer if you used the word could instead of should in that sentence?"

You can't be good at everything. If you are unable to do something that is perfectly normal, ask for help from people that are more experienced in that area. For example, you may need to seek advice from a nutritionist if you want to know more details regarding food.

Self-care involves a lot of areas. Here are a few:

- Rest.
- Time Management.
- Positive self-talk.
- Acceptance of current situation.
- Knowledge that you have the power to change your circumstances.

- Slowing down.
- Asking for support when needed.
- Concentrating on your development and progress.
- Mindfulness/Meditation.
- Being kind, understanding and patient with yourself and others.
- Giving yourself the freedom to adjust at any time to your surround ings.
- Do not let people bully or be rude to you.
- Having ME time. Do something you love.
- Choose what you want.
- Read.
- Take a time out when necessary.
- Surrender but don't give up.
- Set yourself free to do what you want and do it.
- Make a start and don't mind what other people say.
- Have clear determination.

"LAUGHTER
IS WHAT MAKES EVERYTHING BETTER
SO, MAKE SOME TIME FOR IT EVERYDAY"

We all have mental, physical and emotional needs. Here are a few examples of each:

Mental: Reading and learning
Meditation
Socialising
Connecting with others
Petting an animal

Physical: Eating good food.
Get moving. Walking, Tai-chi
Hugs
Massage

Emotional: Creativity
Journalling

Help others

Relax in a warm bath

Balancing everything can be a challenge and staying content is not always easy. There are ways we can help ourselves and when we are aware of these it makes life a lot easier.

In our bodies we all have 4 happy chemicals that help us stay content.

They are as follows:

D. O. S. E.

1. **D** = Dopamine.

This is our pleasure chemical. When we wake up and we have something to look forward to we get excited and we get out of bed easily. Music will help release this, so put on some of your favourite music in the morning and it will lift you.

2 **O** = Oxytocin.

You boost your oxytocin levels from touch and connecting with others. Things like massage, talking, food, kindness and touching someone on the arm are all forms of releasing oxytocin.

3 **S** = Serotonin.

You get this from having a sense of worth, gratitude or feeling united or involved in something. Foods like salmon, green leafy vegetables, spinach, pumpkin chia seed and nuts all help to raise your levels of serotonin.

4 **E** = Endorphins.

When we dance or exercise, we release these chemicals. Even a short 10-minute walk will help.

The best of all is laughter. Even hearing a small child giggling over something silly will lift you and put a smile on your face. This is your Endorphins rising.

What you can do to lift your happy hormones

_____

_____

_____

SHEILA O' HANLON

I had the pleasure of meeting Sheila O' Hanlon about 5 years ago. It has been great fun getting to know her and listening to her amazing advice. We have had Sheila visiting the group in Limerick a few times and she has travelled to other M.E./CFS groups around the country as well. Here is a little piece Sheila put together for you.

I started my Systematic kinesiology training in 2013 and qualified as a practitioner in 2015. I then studied further so I could teach Systematic Kinesiology for the college. After twenty years of high paced, stressful, and physically exhausting jobs I finally found my purpose. To help others to feel better!

I have researched and treated thousands of clients who suffer from fatigue (M.E./CFS and Fibromyalgia)

I have put together a tried and tested list of the most beneficial techniques and lifestyle tweaks that have benefited my clients the most when fighting fatigue!

Please go and visit my YouTube channel for hundreds of health tip videos on exhaustion, digestive issues and much more: Sheila O'Hanlon Kinesiology is my YouTube channel name.

1. Fatigue by definition is lacking energy. Malabsorption in the Small Intestine is always an issue with fatigue clients of mine. A good ionic ZINC supplement heals the mucousy lining of the gut wall, thereby helping the body to be able to absorb more vitamins and minerals from our food. My favourite and the most successful brand is by www.metabolics.com (use the code 180515 for a discount)

2. Burn out – Adrenal fatigue usually precedes fatigue…when your body has given you all it can possibly give you…it literally collapses! Avoiding Caffeine, alcohol, sugary foods, processed nutrient void ready meals, stimulants such as red bull and dramatic people will help you heal more effectively. Stay away from negative, dramatic, and selfish people!

3. Allow yourself time to recover by being kinder to yourself. Take time to do pleasant things, spend time alone in nature for headspace.

4. Learn to say "NO" and have good personal boundaries in place. It's really OK to say no if you don't feel like doing something for others. A lot of my fatigue clients went above and beyond for everyone else, always putting their own needs last…if ever.

5. Drink filtered water every-day to help flush toxins and toxic debris from your organs and colon. Water keeps us alive! At least 1 and half liters per day.

6. Replace Decaf Tea/Coffee…dehydration sets our stress levels higher to begin with.

7. Gentle exercise is better than fast and furious exertion! On a side note when you do occasionally get a burst of energy it is most important to sit with it and allow it to heal and repair your weary body, than waste that precious energy spring cleaning or sorting out the back room wardrobe! Be smart with your energy! Use it wisely. Who cares if the hoovering doesn't get done? what is more urgent? Your healing process or the housework? Let me answer that for you! YOU are the most important thing in your life.

8. Magnesium for cramps is excellent. Also add coriander, parsley, rosemary, thyme, and basil to your diet. All these powerful and tasty herbs are anti Inflammatory by nature.

9. YOU cannot substitute a good night's sleep for anything else…proper repair and regeneration of human cells only happens during sleep. Bed early with total darkness, to block light from the Pineal gland which in turn produces MELATONIN which kick starts repair mode in the body. You can buy eye masks in any chemist or big store.

HOW TO STAY POSITIVE IN A NEGATIVE SITUATION

WHEN YOU FOCUS ON THE GOOD, THE GOOD INCREASES

When you find yourself in a challenging situation ask yourself the following:

- What is it I need at this moment?
- What needs to be done to change this situation?
- Is this really worth getting upset over?
- What have I learnt from this?

REASSURE YOURSELF THAT
THIS TOO WILL PASS
AND BREATHE.

This too shall pass is an expression I use a lot. I used to use this in the bad times to reassure myself that they would not last forever. Now I use this in good times to build wonderful memories. It reminds me to acknowledge, accept and appreciate everything.

Here is a great exercise for reasurrance:

Hold your chin up and your shoulders back. This will instantly influence your mood. Breathe and take a moment. Let go. Next while standing like that say:

I am...............I am

I AM good enough. I AM
I AM clever enough. I AM
I AM beautiful. I AM
I AM able to handle whatever comes my way today. I AM
I AM likeable. I AM
Repeat it until you believe it.
Feel it, really feel it!

On it goes, fill in your own "I am" statements. Write them down and read them every morning and evening. They will give you inner strength. Just make up whatever you wish and put "I am" before and after it to reinforce it. You will find that you do it all the time once you develop the habit.

Tips:
a. Keep it simple, no need to panic. You have time.
b. Try not to overthink the situation.
c. Write down what you need.
d. Be confident in your ability to solve any challenge.
e. Don't be afraid to use your imagination. Look at all the possibilities. This will open the whole situation up.
f. Be gentle and patient with yourself.
ALWAYS!

Patience:

Couldn't we all do with more patience? I know I could! I found dealing with M.E./CFS incredibly challenging and frustrating. I had a lot of resistance for a long time. Limitations can be disruptive to life in general. We can miss out on a lot. Learning to have more patience was a big help to me. I had to learn to adjust and be flexible in my life or I would be extremely unsettled.

To face the reality life has us in now, we need to breathe, take charge, and face up to our situation. Give yourself a couple of minutes each day to just pause. Everyone will differ as our circumstances are unique. If you learn to have more patience it will be worth it! Don't let fear put you off. You're going to have to face whatever the challenge is eventually. The sooner the better as you just cause yourself anxiety by avoiding it. Patience is the key in all you do.

GET UP, GET DRESSED AND GET OUT
BECAUSE SOMETHING WONDERFUL
IS GOING TO HAPPEN WHEN YOU DO

You can always go back to bed at any time if you're not feeling great. I have often had to go back to bed 30 minutes after getting up but been grateful that I got up.

How you hold yourself makes a difference to how you feel, as does how you think and act. Therefore, it is vital to think, be aware and in the moment as much as possible. Have a purpose to your day.

Change: Things are always evolving

Gay Byrne from The Late Late Show, on Irish television, was a big fan of turning expectation into appreciation and would talk about it regularly. If you expect things and you don't get them, then that will cause disappointment. Whereas, if you do things with an open mind with no expectation, then if they work out or not, it makes no difference to you. You get a great buzz when they work out and you will appreciate things even more.

REJECTION

BEHIND EVERY STRONG, INDEPENDENT INDIVIDUAL
LIES SOMEONE WHO HAS FALLEN MANY TIMES AND
HAS HAD TO LEARN HOW TO GET BACK UP AGAIN
AND AGAIN

Handling rejection:
    Be comfortable and confident in your ability. Don't let opinions of others sway you. Don't worry about rejection. If it's meant to be you will get to where you want to go with the right people by your side. To the world you are one person but to one person, you are the world. You won't be everyone's cup of tea, but someone out there will love you and what you do. Be patient and follow your path.

If you reach out to another – you may risk rejection.
If you cry - you may risk being called sentimental.
If you laugh - you may risk being called a fool.
If you open up - you may risk showing your true self.
If you try - you may risk failure.
Don't worry about what is going to happen as most of the time the fear is just that annoying voice in your head trying to put you off.
Just go for it! Be yourself. Say what it is you need to say unapologet-

ically. Don't take yourself too seriously. Laugh at your mistakes and learn from them. It is ok not to be perfect. We will still be learning well into old age.

That makes life exciting.

If you don't jump in and take a chance, you'll never know the wonderful things that are waiting for you. If my husband hadn't asked me to marry him; if he had been too afraid that I would say no, I would not have had the years of adventures we have had together.

If I had let the fear of having a baby overwhelm me, which it almost did - I would not have had the absolute joy in my life that my son, Sam, has given me.

I was watching a programme on television one night about a man who wanted to tell his friend that he loved her. He was too scared of losing their friendship if she rejected him. They remained friends for 40 years and then he plucked up the courage to tell her how he felt. It turned out that she felt the same but was also afraid. They got married a week later as they didn't want to waste any more time. The moral of the story is to grab life by the scruff of the neck and go for it. Just ask, just share, just do whatever it is you want and as long as you're not harming anyone in the process, all will be well.

Ask yourself:

"What exactly is overwhelming me?"

"What's the worst thing that can happen?"

Own that and go for it anyway because, the rewards are so wonderful when you break through your fears.

Give things a try. Don't be stagnant, keep moving forward. Shake things up a bit.

I recently did the 21 days of Abundance Challenge by Deepak Chopra with Eamonn Smith on Facebook. Eamonn has an Advanced Diploma in Mental Health. This challenge involved questions like the following:

• Make a list of 50 people that have influenced your life.

• In what areas of your life would you like to get more abundance?

- Write a letter of gratitude and recognition to a person who hurt you at some point in life.

I tried to do it before but did not finish, so took it on again lately and smashed it. The reason I didn't finish it the first time was because I was afraid of what people would think. I thought things like "What is she doing now? This is silly." This time I just went for it and felt the fear but did it anyway. The feeling of achievement was fabulous, and the exercise benefited me hugely. When I got to the end of the 21 days of Abundance not only did I smash the fear of what others thought but I also learnt to be more accepting and open to the changes around me. I was so happy I did the challenge.

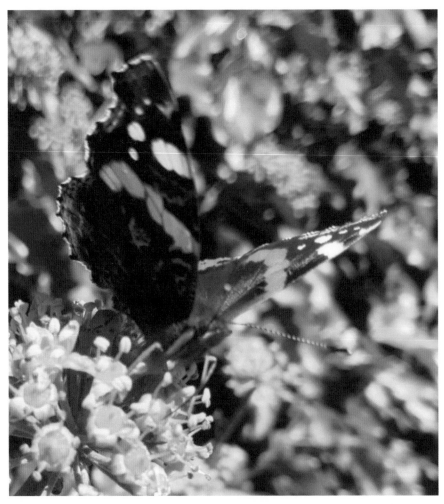

CHOOSE

IF YOU CANNOT DO THE BIG THINGS
DO THE SMALL THINGS IN A GREAT WAY

Will you do it?
Will you make a small change today and act on it?
Are you up for the challenge?
Are you feeling terrible about yourself?
Stop!
Start living a life of self-happiness, where you live up to your potential and dare to follow your dreams. It doesn't matter how small those dreams are as long as you are focussing on what you want.
Stop!
going over all the bad things in your life. Shut the door to the past and focus on the way you want your life to go.

If you think about things too much you will never do anything. Every one of us has millions of thoughts every day and we only act on a small percentage of them.

The 5 second rule
What the hell is this, you ask yourself? Well it's when you get an idea, whatever it may be and before you do anything else you count to

5, and on 5 you act. This way you don't have the time to talk yourself out of it you just say, "Let's go with this and see what happens," then ask yourself:

"What do I need to do now to make this happen"?

Things will start to come into your head, and you will have sorted the next step out and the next and so on. Not every idea will pan out, but you will be more productive than before. Take for example, you love to write poetry, take photos or paint, and one day a thought comes into your mind that makes you think 'I wonder if it's hard to put these together and make a book'? When this happens act quickly and investigate it before the idea drifts by or you convince yourself it's not a good idea. Gather all your notes and get them organised so you can see clearly what you have and then have some fun with it. Remember you don't have to do anything, just play around with the idea and see what happens. See how many poems or paintings etc. you have. Who knows what can happen once you give it a chance.

My son laughs at me because whenever I have a lightbulb moment I write it down straight away because first of all, I will forget it and secondly, I really want to see if it will work. Then I play with the idea on paper with notes of how it could work out, looking at all the possibilities. It stimulates the mind to play around with ideas, no-matter how small. There is no pressure to do anything as you are just investigating. A couple of mine have come about. This book is one of them.

One day Sam and I were chatting, and he casually mentioned that I should write a book as I am very passionate about helping others to improve their quality of life. I played around with it for a few days and before I knew it, I had designed how I wanted it to look and had named 10 of the chapters I would put in. It all just started to flow out of me. It was amazing how it all came about. Later that same week a good friend of mine Pat McCurtain said the same thing to me out of the blue. I knew then I had to do this no matter how long it took me.

I have come across a lot of people who are starting to believe in themselves. One person I know who has this condition, has written a book on poems, another does fabulous illustrations. One of my friends who is in a wheelchair because of this condition, has lost 6 stone over

4 years. He told me he altered a few things in his diet, e.g. portion size, cut out sweet things and lowered carbohydrates. Amazing!

It doesn't matter how big or small your goal is as long as what you decide to put your mind to ends up with the desired results.

It can be fifteen minutes meditation for thirty days or a ten-minute walk daily if you're up to it. Everything is an achievement. Just enjoy the journey.

Ask yourself:

Do you sometimes feel like you cannot ask for what you genuinely want or say no because you fear being rejected?

Do you feel like no matter how well you do things; you are still not good enough or happy on the inside?

Do you feel like you are not someone who could have or deserve what you want in life?

Do you feel discouraged?

Do you think you'd have more success in life if you were happier on the inside?

You can improve all these feelings. Make little changes now! Choose what you want to adjust. Your thoughts have a huge part to play in everything. If your thoughts are off, everything will be out of balance.

The 5 second rule will sort some of these out and acceptance of your particular situation sorts the rest.

It took me a while into my journey with M.E./CFS to learn to accept the situation I was in. I got help and everything became so much easier. I wish I could have learnt all this a lot quicker. That's why I'm writing this book so you can get the tips and tricks now and do for yourself what I couldn't. This will release a lot of pressure. Now I am not saying to give up. Far from it! I am simply saying to learn to accept your limits as they are for the moment and agree to keep working on improving your quality of life as best you can.

You can find ways of doing things by adjusting your plans. For example, if you want to go somewhere and you're afraid it will be too much of a challenge for you, plan it out. Have cat naps and spread everything out. Things that took you one day to do before might have to be spread out over three days, so you don't get too fatigued.

My son moved to England when he was only sixteen and I was determined to go to see him, so I booked flights and arranged accommodation. My husband and I came up with a plan. I took it easy for a few days prior to leaving, pacing myself very strictly. I went to bed extra early the night before and slept in the car while Jim drove us to the airport. Then when we arrived at the hotel I lay down and rested. The following morning, we went to see Sam. In the afternoon I slept while Sam went off with his Dad and then later all of us would get a bite to eat and catch up.

When you have obstacles in your life you can work your way around them at whatever pace suits you.

LOW SELF-ESTEEM AND HOW TO DEAL WITH IT

YOU CAN BE HAPPIER AND MORE SATISFIED IN YOUR LIFE, NO MATTER WHAT YOUR SITUATION IT'S ALL ABOUT HOW YOU LOOK AT THINGS

Low self-esteem is caused by looking at yourself in an overly critical manner and completely ignoring your positive qualities. If you don't address the issue you could be extremely unhappy. You may find yourself looking inward with strong negative emotions and this is very unpleasant and not recommended. You can see it in people by their body language and how they act. They feel inadequate and deflated and this will come across in the language they use.

It is quite easy to let this condition or life in general, get you down. I was terrified of depression for years so kept a close eye on my moods. I worked hard at being positive. I finally made a breakthrough when I was talking to a friend of mine who told me to be realistically positive as it is exhausting trying to be positive all the time. It also leads to denial. He explained that if the day is not going according to plan, acknowledge it and accept the real situation. Then move on and do what you can to turn it around. Take for example, you get up and you feel awful. Next thing you know you spill your tea and get jam on your clothes. Then you get a call from someone who is not in good form and next thing you know you're bawling your eyes out and just want to scream! There are two things you can do here. Stay fed up and go on with your day in terrible form, trying to be positive and pretending all is well. Or you can acknowledge that the day has been disastrous so far and accept it. Decide consciously that you are going to do something about it, by facing the day head on. Set yourself free from the avoidance. It's good to be positive but you must be careful not to avoid the reality of life as well.

Let's look at what you can do to help yourself:

The good news is lots can be done to turn things around. I want to discuss where self-esteem comes from first. In my case it was embedded at an early age from being told by teachers and the nuns at school that I wasn't very bright. I learnt later in life that this was not the case. I was a little free spirited, basically a happy child who liked to fly around having fun. Now this didn't go down well with the nuns as you can imagine; they liked to control everything, and I didn't really fit into their ways. So, early emotional conditioning is mostly to blame for my low self-esteem.

I once had a nun tell me in front of a classroom of students that she couldn't believe how stupid I was. This stuck with me for an exceptionally long time. As it turned out, that was a load of rubbish as later in life when I went to night school I did very well in my exams, proving to myself that with a bit of persistence and sticking to things a bit longer, I could get there and figure things out. When I lived in Vancouver, I was doing a computer course. There were several people in the class, and you worked individually. There was a part of the programme that I found particularly challenging. After seven attempts I finally got my head around it. Mary sitting across from me picked it up on the third attempt. Some of us need more time to figure it out. That's okay. If my self-esteem were in the gutter as it had been before I would have given up much earlier and not figured it out at all. Instead I stuck with it and persisted again and again until I got there. When we are faced with the challenges of this condition it will knock us down repeatedly. We must persist and keep moving forward believing in ourselves that someday we will have a better quality of life. That day is now. If you use the tools I have in this book, I hope you will find life much easier to manage. You have got this far, made it through all the ups and downs this condition has thrown at you, and you are still here reading this book. That shows that you want to make changes to your life. If you make the changes and tweak things just a little, you will notice improvements.

What can you do?
Start with observing your thoughts. When you start negative self-talk, stop yourself right away.
Stop thinking about what you can't do and think about what you want to do based on what you can do.
Next ask yourself:
"What do I need to do?"
Your mind is a mechanism built to adapt to new situations. You just need to ask it questions to activate it.
Once you open up your mind to receive, the answers will come. Just relax. If you change your situation, by creating a new one, the one you want will manifest itself. Your brain will automatically rewire itself to understand the new stream of information.

What you think about you bring about
The mind is like a magnet. It attracts what you think about. If you think of all the possibilities it will bring more and more ideas to mind. If you think of obstacles it will bring you more of those also. I know what I would choose.

The cells in your body react to everything that your mind says. So be incredibly careful about what you think and say. Not only that but it will wreak havoc with your immune system, and you don't want that.

HAPPINESS CAN BE FOUND EVEN IN THE DARKEST OF TIMES, IF YOU ONLY REMEMBER TO TURN ON THE LIGHT
Albus Dumbledore

CONFIDENCE

IT IS CONFIDENCE IN OUR OWN ABILITY, MIND AND BODY THAT ALLOWS US TO MOVE FORWARD

We were not born with a lack of confidence. Someone once asked me "Was your son self-conscious when he learnt to walk or did he just do it?" The answer was he just did it. He fell a few times but got right back up again and eventually he got the hang of it. He did not care what anyone thought or who was looking at him. This is because we are not self-conscious as children. We unfortunately learn this as we grow up. If we can manage our fear and anxiety around what others think and say, we will reduce them as our confidence will rise.

Start by changing the picture in your head. We are back to your thoughts. What others think of you is not important as they do not really know you. Know that what you are doing is right for you and stick with it. You have a voice and what you have to say is important to you so say whatever you need to say. Be confident in your abilities. Know that you are intelligent.

Tweak the things that come to mind if they are not serving you. You need to do what is in your own best interest.

Fear can be managed if you change the story of what is happening. Get excited about what you are facing. Enjoy the task.

Compliment yourself regularly so you build your self-esteem and in turn your confidence will rise.

Tell yourself what you want to hear. Choose to do things you really want to do e.g. feel good, feel enough, feel strong. Use the I am exercise: I am beautiful. I am kind. I am resilient. I am confident. I can do things to help myself.

Low self-confidence is a challenge, but you can improve it so that you can feel good about yourself again and get on with life. Take charge as you can control this.

People can be hard on themselves. This is unfortunate. Things get difficult and we can't be strong all the time. That's okay. Don't be afraid to ask for help. I did and it changed my life completely. So, reach out and ask for help and get the advice needed. I bet you will be pleasantly surprised how wonderful people can be. Just take the chance.

Once I started to accept my situation, things changed for me. I never gave up, but I took a more realistic approach to where I was at that point in life and what this condition was doing to me. I started to tweak parts of my life and I took on a "let's do this" attitude. Sometimes it's hard to motivate yourself and you need to give yourself a gentle nudge and encourage yourself. I'm not saying this will be easy, but it will be worth your while.

"YOU CAN DO THIS! LIFE WILL CHALLENGE YOU BUT YOU HAVE COME THIS FAR SO DON'T STOP NOW. YOU CAN HELP YOURSELF THROUGH LIFE'S UPS AND DOWNS BY BELIEVING IN YOURSELF! BE CONFIDENT IN YOUR ABILITY TO DO WHATEVER IT IS YOU CHOOSE."

This will be a new routine and you will be mentally stronger every day and before you know it, hey presto, you will notice the changes.

It is a lifestyle change, and you will notice dips but that's okay. The small things you achieve will start to add up and you will become stronger as your confidence increases. You are so worth it and the sooner you realise how special you are, the better. Take everything slow and steady.

Small things like criticism, failure or problems will not bother you as much as they used to. You won't react the same. You will be calmer and more confident because you know you can deal with them calmly. Remember you can change anything. Things can constantly be tweaked until they are to your liking.

STOP SEEKING APPROVAL FROM OTHERS.
BE CONFIDENT ENOUGH TO KNOW
YOU ARE VERY CAPABLE YOU DON'T
NEED OTHERS APPROVAL.

Try these:
• **Handle the criticism** and negativity in a more understanding and level-headed way. Stay grounded. Breathe. Come from a place of love, not hate.
• **Stop comparing yourself** and your life to other people. We all have stuff, simply different stuff. You never know what is going on in others' lives. It may look perfect, but you can be sure things are not always greener on the other side.
• **Nothing is perfect** and perfectionism will only drive you crazy. We are all human. We all make mistakes. Trying to be perfect leads to stress and anxiety and it is very tiring.
• **Trust yourself** to be able to handle life and make the important decisions.
• **Acknowledge your weaknesses.** We can't be good at everything, even if we want to be. Know your strengths and keep building them while working on your weak areas and all will be fine.
• **Let your inner voice** be kind.
• **Be Kind and compassionate** towards yourself and others. Understand that people hide the hard times and will only open up when truly understood.

Name 3 things that make you feel confident.
1.
2.
3.

Start introducing more of these activities into your life.

A LITTLE SPARK OF KINDNESS CAN PUT BURSTS OF SUN-
SHINE INTO SOMEONE'S DAY. STAY STRONG AS YOU ARE
THE LIGHT IN SOMEONE ELSE'S LIFE.

Believe in yourself
1. Investigate all the possibilities that are open to you.
2. Have no fear. Fear will mess everything up for you.
3. Be confident in your own ability. Know what you are good at and keep improving. Houses need good foundations and so do we.
4. Eliminate self-doubt.
5. Think about all your options.

Take a moment, breathe, and create space. Move forward in a calm state. A tense mind and body are not going to do you any good because you are not going to be able to think straight.

Control the controllables
You can't control everything, and this is very important to acknowledge. We have control over what we say, our behaviour, our diet, exercise, rest, goals, stress, anxiety, actions, mistakes etc. and what we decide to do with them. We can't control other people's actions, what they say or think or feel. Their beliefs, ideas and opinions are not ours to change. We are all free to do what we want and that's what makes life interesting. Simply agree to differ if you don't agree. It's just an opinion, it doesn't mean it's right. Don't let other opinions damage your confidence.

These are all things we need to let go of and not try to control as they are not our responsibility.

Don't waste your time and energy trying to change others. Not everyone will be on your side and that's ok.

We are all entitled to our opinion. If we all had the same views and opinions life would be very boring. We all think we are right. So just move on. Don't upset yourself over things you can't control.

I was listening to an interview with bestselling author Steve Cavanagh. He said he had over 150 rejections for his first book. The interviewer asked him "How did you keep going after so many rejections?" and Steve replied "I knew I was going to get there in the end. I could feel it, and nobody could put me off." Now that's confidence!

As Forrest Gump says,
"MY MOMMA ALWAYS SAID,
LIFE IS LIKE A BOX OF CHOCOLATES.
YOU NEVER KNOW WHAT
YOU'RE GONNA GET"

That's what makes life fun. Challenges make us stronger!
It all starts in the BRAIN. If you genuinely believe you are something, you must embody that feeling. Say you went into a coma and then woke up. Say you were told you were a dancer before you lost your memory. Do you think you'd hold yourself differently, conduct yourself differently, and have a different outlook on life? As opposed to being told you were a construction worker?
This is a story about the mind. I realise we have M.E./CFS and are physically limited but the point I'm making here is regarding mindset. It's all about your outlook and your thoughts.
How do each of these following sentences feel?
"I believe I am the best actor in the world", versus "I hope I am the best actor in the world".
Your tone of voice will be different for each. The first quote is far more convincing, yes?
The brain is like a circuit. If you have the right wiring, you'll work better. Your words are extremely important. The brain will believe what you tell it. The story you tell yourself is critical.
Everyone has doubts. Don't dwell on these. It gets you nowhere. Flip the script to what you want it to be.
It's all about how you handle the negative thoughts in that moment. Change to stronger positive thoughts that allow you to move on and get what you want.
Have confidence in yourself and believe you can do this.

Confidence fluctuates all the time. How you handle the knocks, and the comments will make a difference.

Internal conflicts happen all the time, but you need to handle the situation, and trust in yourself that you can do this. You are strong.

See things differently. Look at the end line, the result you're after. What you want and believe, you will get. Want to do this. Be excited. Have your plan made out and all will work in your favour. It has before and it will again. Step by step you will get to the end line and achieve your desired goal.

It's good to have an accountability buddy. I started daily meditation to keep me calm. My buddy checked in on me to see if I was sticking to my plan and this kept me on track. You can do a task together and help each other out so that you stay on course. I found it a great help.

Everybody has it in them to do whatever they wish, no matter how big or small your goal.

But will you? Do you want it bad enough? Are you willing to do what it takes?

For example, will you eat healthier and put good food into your body so that you are giving it the nutrition it needs?

Will you observe your thoughts and inner voice so that your emotions are more balanced? If you can do these few things you're on the road to a more content life.

Take a good look at what you want to alter. There is no time like the present. Write down one thing right now that you want to change for the better. Don't put it off any longer. You will thank yourself later. It's like building a house, one brick at a time.

It won't always be easy as you are going to have to make choices. It takes time. You have time. If it's important enough, you'll make time. Follow your heart. Feel it! Want it with every fibre of your being. You may stumble but you will get up. You always do. You are stronger than you give yourself credit for. Look at your past and everything you have got through and you are still here. That's success. That's will power. That's resilience. Sometimes you lose, that's life. Sometimes you win, that's sweet.

Remember:
- Make up your own mind.
- Take action, stop talking about it.
- Take the first step.

It will take self-discipline and little pushes to move and make the right choices, but it will be worth it.
- Trust that everything will take its course and will be what it will be. Let go and let the universe take care of it.
- If you are not happy do something about it. Take action and change things up.
- Tell someone today that you appreciate them.
- Stay foolish. Don't take yourself too seriously.
- Have a dream, what is it?
- Feel the fear and go for it.
- Resist the temptation to criticise.
- Take charge of your thoughts. STOP negative self-talk.
- Stay focussed. There will be setbacks. That's life
- Energy drainers must go. Be around people that nourish you.
- Feed your brain daily.

STAY STRONG, YOU ARE RESILIENT. LOOK AT EVERYTHING YOU'VE FACED, ALL THE ISSUES YOU'VE SORTED. YOU CAN DO THIS!

COMFORT ZONE

IF IT DOESN'T CHALLENGE YOU IT DOESN'T CHANGE YOU

Are you doing all you can do to help yourself? What small changes can you make? Start working on getting out of your comfort zone. Try new things. You may ask,
"How do I get out of my comfort zone"?

Well the answer is, very gently. Go little by little. There is no rush, take it at whatever pace suits you. It's important to work on it daily by manoeuvering how you approach situations in your life. Try new things every opportunity you get. Don't overthink things as you will talk yourself out of it if you don't act quickly. Small steady progress.

You will see the rings on the inside of the trunk if you look at a freshly cut down tree.

Each ring represents a year in the life of the tree. You will notice there is a space between each ring. If you start in the centre of the circle of rings, you will notice they are closely together and as you work your way out to the outside by the bark, the rings become further apart. Now imagine you are in the centre, the core of the tree, and each ring is your new level of comfort. You will have to push yourself a little and be brave each time you move from one ring to the next. Each ring represents you moving on and progressing out of your comfort zone into new levels. At each ring you will open up and become bigger, stronger, and braver as you move from ring to ring.

I started doing this back in 2007. I was asked to read out a list of names at a gathering. I had a massive fear of reading in public. I said yes before I knew where I was. I was embarrassed to say no, so I took the plunge. I did it and got through it, as terrified as I was. That was the first step for me in tackling my fear and getting out of my comfort zone. I was petrified beforehand but I got through it, and it was ok. Slowly but surely after that I did little talks, introducing someone, e.g. Dr. Ross Vallings to a crowd, or announcing upcoming events at a coffee morning. Small things that took no more than a few minutes. Now I know I can do up to twenty minutes talking on a topic in front of an audience. I still have to do one more thing which is, read in public. This will be the big test. I know I will do it someday. When I do, I will imagine touching the bark and smiling as this will be my task of public speaking completed. I can then build on it with confidence, knowing I can do it. I use this exercise to face all my obstacles. I am looking forward to when this book is published as I will be able to imagine touching the bark again and I will smile a big smile.

Pick a topic that you want to achieve and start small. Step out of your comfort zone today and grow. Set an intention in place. Write it down here:

Today I am going to…

I find it incredibly relaxing to walk through wooded areas and watch the trees dance in the wind. It's so freeing and hypnotic.

APPRECIATION AND GRATITUDE
CAN ATTRACT GOOD THINGS
INTO YOUR LIFE.

Name 3 things you are grateful for
1.
2.
3.

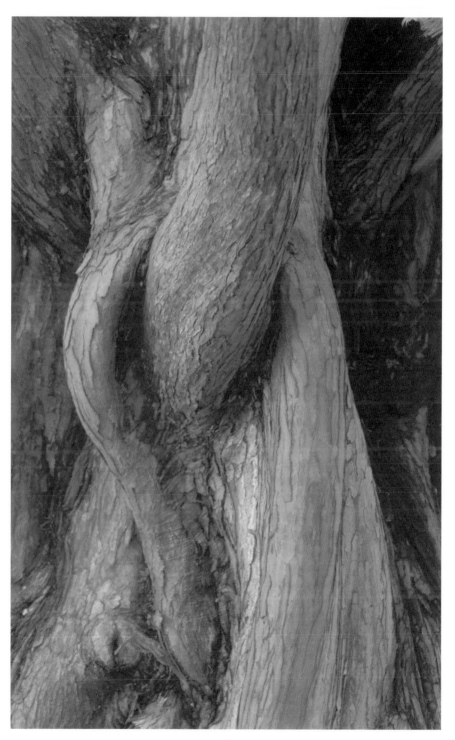

CHANGE

"THE SMALLEST ACT OF KINDNESS IS WORTH
MORE THAN THE GREATEST INTENTION."
Kahlil Gibran

You have a choice with every situation. How you choose will depend on the level of confidence you have in your own ability. This will differ for each of us. I believe we deserve the respect of others. Changes will have to be made. We need to be brave and set boundaries, so you feel safe. Decide what is best for you and choose it daily. Every minute of the day when you are faced with a decision ask yourself:
"What do I want?"
"What changes can be made here?"
"What do I need to do right now to get it?"
"How will that make me feel?"

Be aware and mindful when you do this. Don't let anything distract you. Place your full attention on the task at hand.

Find ways to be mindful and present. This will balance your mind and body. The more relaxed you are the more changes you will make.

One of my favourite sayings, that I have clung to over the past fifteen years or so is from Zig Ziglar. He was a motivational speaker/Author who died back in 2012. Zig would talk about the three Cs in life: CHOICE, CHANCE AND CHANGE.

When you make a choice, you take a chance, and things will change. If you do this, things will happen and if you don't life will never change. This has helped me on my road as I revisit it regularly to remind myself to shake things up.

Choosing the right options was vital in my journey with this condition. I had to make lots of changes. There was a couple of times when I could have very easily gone down the wrong path and it took willpower and thank goodness, I made the right choices – e.g.

1. I choose not to let this condition make me bitter.
2. I choose to look on food as a form of medicine.
3. I choose to focus on others.

Sharing what I have learnt to those who want to hear it. Police your thoughts and erase and delete the ones you don't want and keep the ones you do. Remind yourself that you are good enough and if anyone tries to tell you differently, remember that it is their opinion, and you are agreeing to differ. We all have opinions. It doesn't mean they are right. They are just opinions.

Don't waste time. Choose wisely because you can feel better and improve your quality of life if you do. Who you spend your time with has a huge effect on your wellbeing.

Notice how you feel when people talk to you, happy, sad, angry, uplifted etc. If you don't like it, you have the power to change it. Be around people that lift you up not bring you down! Life is too short, make the most of every day. If someone doesn't respect you and you don't like it, then do something about it!

Be determined. Don't be afraid. Time is precious, waste it wisely. Life is not always easy, but we can always do something to make our situation better. Attitude is important. There is a story about two men in a hospital room and one of them is blind. It goes like this:

One man was allowed to sit up in his bed for an hour each afternoon to help drain the fluid from his lungs. His bed was next to the room's only window. The other man had to spend all his time flat on his back.

They spoke of their wives and families, their homes, their jobs, their in-

volvement in the military service, holidays etc.

Every afternoon, when the man in the bed next to the window could sit up, he would pass the time by describing to his roommate all the things he could see outside the window.

The man in the other bed began to love those one hour periods where his world would be broadened and enlivened by all the activity and colour of the world outside. The window overlooked a park with a lovely lake. Ducks and swans played on the water while children sailed their model boats. Young lovers walked arm in arm amidst flowers of every colour and a fine view of the city skyline could be seen in the distance. As the man by the window described all this in exquisite details, the man on the other side of the room would close his eyes and imagine this picturesque scene. One warm afternoon, the man by the window described a parade passing by. Although the other man could not hear the band, he could see it clearly in his mind as it was being described in clear descriptive words.

After months of this a nurse arrived one morning to bring water to the men. The man by the window was lifeless as he had passed peacefully in his sleep. This saddened her as she rang to arrange for him to be taken away.

The other man in the room was moved over by the window. Slowly and painfully he propped himself up on one elbow to take his first look at the real world outside. He strained to slowly turn to look out the window beside his bed. It faced a blank wall. The man asked the nurse what could have compelled his deceased roommate who had described such beautiful things outside the window. The nurse informed him that the man was blind. She said, "Perhaps he just wanted to brighten your day and encourage you".

I love this story. It just shows how you look at the world can alter everything. You have a choice. There is enormous pleasure and happiness to be had by helping others and making them smile.

One of my favourite things to do is to make others smile. It warms my heart. Despite our own situation. We all have challenges and sadness in our lives but how we manage them will make a tremendous difference to our quality of life.

Happiness when shared is a joy. It is contagious so spread it far and wide. Look at the things in life that money can't buy like, love, integrity, patience, manners, morals, respect, character, friendship, loyalty, time, intimacy, and empathy.

Today is here now and it is a gift. It will be gone before you know it so enjoy it as much as you can. I realise we are limited but there are things we can do, so focus on those. Be present and in the moment as much as you can.

By adjusting your outlook and changing your attitude you will notice an instant shift. Enjoy!

Spend time developing yourself. Work on yourself, little by little, always moving forward. Try things out.

It takes time. Making good habits and choosing wisely is time well spent.

WHAT YOU THINK ABOUT YOU BRING ABOUT.

BE OPEN
LOVE OFTEN
EAT HEALTHY
MOVE MORE
WORRY LESS
THINK POSITIVELY
STAY STRONG
BE HAPPY
SING

Ask yourself:

What are you most proud of in your life? Focus on you, and your achievements.

List 3 things

1.

2.

3.

How do you feel after answering this question?

Pause and feel how your heart feels. Is it like its expanding / growing in your chest?

What emotions come up?

Is that a smile I see?

As time goes by you will become aware of different things that put a smile on your face. Make note of them and introduce more of them into your daily/weekly routine.

Taking photos is one of my favourite things to do. I carry my camera with me most times now when I go for some fresh air as there is always something that draws me in, and I just have to take a photograph of it. Autumn is spectacular with all the rustic colours of the leaves and flowers, so breathtakingly beautiful.

I am no expert by any means. I just like to click and go. Usually by the end of a day when I look back over the photos, I find at least a couple that make me smile and then I am happy.

It does not take much energy and the joy it brings is enormous.

What could you get excited about in your life right now? You can change your state of mind in seconds. When you discover what makes you tick, it will alter your life forever. Try different things until you feel joy. Time will fly by. Sing a song, put on music, dance, if only for a minute, call a friend etc.

> "REAL CHANGE, ENDURING CHANGE,
> HAPPENS ONE STEP AT A TIME"
> *Justice Ruth Bader Ginsburg*

Pay attention to the sounds around you as they will trigger memories from the past. I was sitting on a wall near my house, waiting for my son the other day. We walked up to get some milk. It was a glorious evening as the sun was cooling off and the temperature was very pleasant. As I was sitting on the wall, watching life go by, enjoying the moment to just chill, a boy passed by on his bike and as he did I heard the clicking of the gears as he adjusted his speed upwards. I immediately went back in time to when I used to ride my bike, more than twenty years ago in Vancouver. I could feel the joy of speeding along the coast road with the views and smells of the ocean on my righthand side. My gears clicking as I gained momentum and the feeling of joy, confidence, excitement, and freedom was heavenly. I could feel the strength in my legs as they did what I asked of them. What a glorious feeling that was. Gliding along with the wind blowing through my hair. Free as a bird.

The point of this story is to remind you to listen to the sounds and pay attention to the feelings that arise when memories of joy, good times and happiness pop up. Savour these moments and if you like jot them down when you get home so that next time you are feeling grey, you can look at your note book and read what brought a smile to your face in the past.

What would you like to change in your life? Take a good look. What do you want? Write it down. Make a simple realistic plan. What is in your life that gives you a sense of meaning and purpose? Find it! Work on it. It can save your life.

Name 3 things you could change that would benefit you:
1.
2.
3.

What makes your heart sing?

What brightens your day?

OUTLOOK IS A CHOICE
ATTITUDE IS A CHOICE.
HAPPINESS IS A CHOICE.
OPTIMISM IS A CHOICE.
COMPASSION IS A CHOICE
KINDNESS IS A CHOICE.
GIVING IS A CHOICE.
RESPECT IS A CHOICE.
WHAT CHOICES WILL YOU MAKE?
CHOOSE WISELY.

DETACHMENT &
OBSERVATION

YOU CAN'T CONTROL
THE ACTIONS AND WORDS
OF OTHERS

This is a very powerful tool to use. It gives you a different perspective on any situation.

Association v disassociation

The easiest way to describe these is to use examples. Association: This is when you are being dragged into something and you lose complete control of the situation and are completely submerged in it. An example would be when you have an argument with someone, and it gets heated and you end up saying all sorts of things you regret afterwards. All reason goes out the window.

Disassociation on the other hand is when you distance yourself from the situation at hand and become detached and are emotionally intact.

Imagine yourself on a balcony and you're watching two other people arguing down below. Your emotions are intact. You are not part of the conversation, so you don't react, just observe. You are not out of control and your breathing is regular. You are clear and calm about what you are seeing.

Practice this while in conversations with people who are challenging. Breathe and ground yourself. Listen without judgement or reaction. Step back in your head so you are disassociated like you were when you stood on the balcony watching from above. Keep a logical mind. Stay calm so you can think straight.
It takes time to master and you will not succeed every time. When you do, it's a great feeling and immensely powerful.

You're in an observing mode. No matter how excited the other person gets, (and they will react) just breathe and step back mentally, not physically. Stay grounded - your thoughts will remain clear.

It is all about setting boundaries to protect yourself. The new you does not listen to confrontation and belittling comments. People will see that you aren't reacting and move onto someone else.

As you get stronger and more confident you will start to be able to express yourself and say what you want. When you are clear and calm people will take you seriously.

BREATHE AND TAKE A MINUTE
BE PRESENT AND GROUNDED
STEP BACK IN YOUR HEAD
THEN TALK

Ripples
"You can make a difference in someone's life, but know this, not only will you impact their life, but you also impact everyone they meet as well! It doesn't matter how small the act is, it ripples on and on. So, start a ripple today and smile in the knowing that it will go on and on".

Ask yourself:
What do I want to change in my life?
What do I love doing? Make a list.
What do I want to overcome?
What are my strengths?

What do I need to work on?

What type of person do I want to be?

How do I go about getting there?

What is my first step going to be?

Are there things in my life that are not serving me?

Can I adjust certain aspects of my life to benefit me?

What makes me unhappy, lonely, inadequate, sad, fearful, joyful?

What am I going to do about changing the things I don't like into things I do like? Talk to some friends and hear their suggestions. Ask for help. Set boundaries.

Communication is the key!

YOU HAVE A CHOICE TO DECIDE
WHAT IT IS YOU WANT

The f word

If you are excited about something, give it a try. HAVE SOME FUN. Nothing will happen until you decide to switch into gear. What is the worst that can happen? It is not the end of the world if it doesn't come to anything. At least you tried. You are stronger than you give yourself credit for. Look what you have accomplished so far in your life and be proud of yourself.

Keep telling yourself you deserve the good things in your life. You have it in you to do what needs to be done to get them. Have you been putting something off for a while? Do you want to get more organised or sort out all your clothes, garden, art, files, poetry etc.

For example, what happens in an emergency?

You do what needs to be done and you do not even think about it, you spring into action and you get through it. You did not have time to think it over, you act because you have to! If you could bring a little of that motivation into your life, the not overthinking, the just doing part, you would benefit a lot.

I had to make a phone call to ask someone for something. I do not usually like asking for things because of the fear of them saying no.

This is where I had to give myself a little push and just do it. Not to overthink it just pick up the phone and dial!

Fear is good to a certain extent if you manage it and don't let it stop you getting what you want. A certain amount of fear will motivate you. It gets you prepared.

"TAKE ACTION BECAUSE SOMETHING WONDERFUL HAPPENS EVERY TIME YOU DO!".

What do you want to do today?
Which invitation do you want to accept?
Hang in there. It is astonishing how short a time it can take for good things to happen.

YOU WILL GROW THROUGH
WHAT YOU GO THROUGH.

STOP COMPARING

BE YOURSELF. YOU ARE UNIQUE

Constantly comparing your life and yourself to other people is a dangerous game that only brings unhappiness.
We may have a habit of comparing cars, houses, jobs, shoes, money, relationships, etc. This can create a lot of negative feelings inside and we become jealous and unhappy. Set your own path.

Here are tips that may help

Be kind
The way you think and behave towards others has a big effect on how you think and behave about yourself.

If you judge people harshly you are more likely going to judge yourself the same way. Be more understanding and kind to other people. Help them, and you will be more kind and helpful towards yourself.

Treat others the same way as you would want to be treated. Be kind to people. What you give out swings back at you so think before acting.
Focus your mind on helping others. Judging yourself and others is

not healthy. Focus on the positive things in yourself and others. There is good in everyone.

You will become more content with yourself and others in your world if you take on a more compassionate outlook.

Don't compare

You are unique. Believe in yourself always. There is no one else in the world quite like you. Even identical twins are different in some ways. Comparing yourself to others is futile. It is like comparing apples with oranges. Have people around you that you learn from and that you look up to.

It's not a contest

Enjoy what you choose to do. Be the best you can be at whatever you choose. There will always be people that are better than you at something. If we were all the same life would be very boring.

Sort out your inner voice

Stop the negative chatter in your head. It is hard enough to deal with other's negative language without adding to it yourself. Bringing others down to build yourself up does not work. You feel worse. Talk back to your internal critic. Change the voice in your head to a loving one.

Be grateful

Create a habit of gratitude and give thanks for everything you have. Look at your strengths and feed them. Watch them grow and be happy. See all the people around you that helped you get where you are today. Look how far you have come. Picture all the wonderful experiences you have had. Cherish them and relive them in your mind. They will make you smile and feel incredibly grateful. You have progressed so far, and you have achieved so much. Reset your goals and move on. Put one foot in front of the other and move forward at your own pace.

The habit of being grateful for the things around you has the benefit of creating joy, happiness, appreciation and kindness towards yourself and others. You will start to observe your reality in a whole new light. You will see how far you have come, and the obstacles you have overcome. It is a glorious feeling.

Be happy with yourself.

Please see chapter on Gratitude on page 79, for more information.

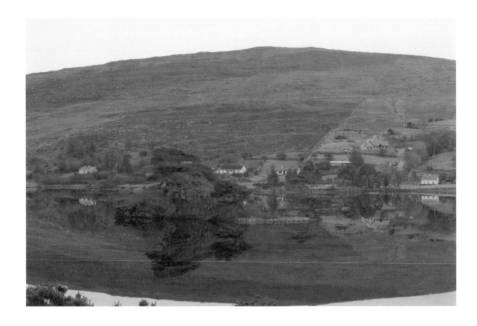

ALWAYS SEND OUT GOOD VIBES
AS THOSE VIBES WILL COME BACK TO YOU TENFOLD
IN UNEXPECTED WONDERFUL WAYS

Here is a little story I heard some time ago, that helped me a lot. I hope it does the same for you.

It is a story about an unusual friendship between a mouse and a whale.

Once there was a mouse, who wanted to build a boat. Eventually, he did just that. When he had finished, he took his boat out on the sea. He was so happy he forgot about the time and drifted far from the shore. Suddenly he realised and tried to turn the boat around, but the winds had grown extraordinarily strong and he began to panic. Just as he was beginning to feel he was in real trouble a wave came and the mouse got thrown overboard.

Suddenly he felt something happen. He seemed to be lifting. Startled by all this he looked around frantically only to realise that a whale had come to his rescue. The mouse now sat on the whale's back. With a big smile on his face, the mouse got up and started running up and down the whale's back.

After a while they reached an Island and the mouse hopped off the whale's back and they said their goodbyes. The mouse lived on the Island and was very happy with his new life.

One day when the mouse was playing on the beach, he noticed something in the distance. As it approached, he recognised it was his friend the whale. He was in trouble. He had come too close to the shore and got stuck in the shallow waters and needed help. The mouse called two of his friends who were elephants, and they pushed the whale to safety.

The whale and the mouse were left in a place where they had to say goodbye again. Although they were sad and both cried, they knew they would be friends forever and remain in each other's hearts always.

I found this very comforting as I have friends and family that are far away and some that are gone for good, but I know they will be in my heart forever and ever.

MAY YOU HAVE
ALL THE JOY
YOUR HEART CAN HOLD

ADJUST YOUR OUTLOOK

BELIEVE AND YOU WILL ACHIEVE

DON'T GIVE UP!
ADJUST THE PLAN AND TRY AGAIN.
HOW YOU LOOK AT THINGS MAKE ALL THE
DIFFERENCE TO THE SITUATION YOU ARE IN.

Sleep and why it is important
If you are tired everything looks different, and not for the better.
Your whole outlook on life changes after a good night's sleep.
It is vital for you to get a good night's sleep, we all know that.
Why is it so important?
What does it do?
How can we improve our sleep?

Firstly, sleep allows your body to heal and repair. Sleep is the only time your body gets to clear away dead cells and repair the damaged ones. If this doesn't happen then it leads to unforeseen consequences.
The good news is that we can improve our sleep by making a few simple adjustments to our evening routine.

1. Turn off all electrical devices an hour or two before bed. This

includes TV, laptops, phones, etc.

2. Make sure your pillows are comfortable.

3. Declutter your bedroom.

4. Have gentle lighting in your bedroom.

5. Preferably, do not have a TV in your bedroom.

6. Have comfortable bedding.

7. Listening to gentle music before you go to sleep helps enormously.

8. Try not to drink too much after 6pm

I usually sip a half a mug of warm milk with nutmeg and honey, as it's a natural sleeping aid. Sip away on that an hour or two before bed.

9. Magnesium has proven to be effective as well. You can have it in a little water, or you can put Epsom salts into your bath before bed.

Stress also impacts on our sleep. If your thoughts are causing you stress, remind yourself this is not the time to deal with those issues and that tomorrow is another day. You can deal with them then. There may be nothing that can be done late at night so park your thoughts for the night and replace them with more pleasant ones. Know that this is the time to relax and drift off into a lovely peaceful sleep. Go to nice places in your mind. I go to beautiful gardens and beaches. I fill my head with relaxing visualisations.

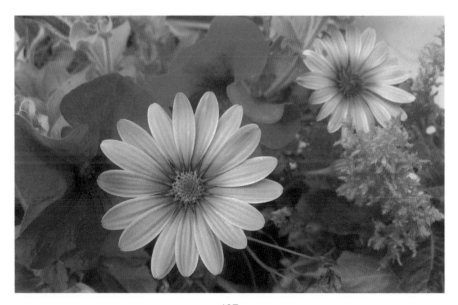

Embrace a new day:

Every day is a new start and can feel good from the get-go. Start by taking a deep breath in and letting it go. Do this 3 times. Believe that this is going to be a good day and decide that nobody is going to upset you today. They are not going to steal your good mood. You can handle anything that pops up. You are very capable. It's important to be grounded. Stand up and make sure your feet are firmly on the ground. Breathe in and out of your nose and visualise roots from your feet going into the ground.

If you can do five minutes of meditation that would be wonderful to set your mood for the day.

I usually try visualisation each morning. Sometimes I see myself by the sea and other times I travel around in my head on a magic carpet to different parts of the world, e.g. the Grand Canyon. It's so much fun. It puts me in a good mood and ready to face the world. Promise yourself you're not going to let anyone, or anything, ruin your day or take your good mood away. If somebody challenges you, just repeat in your head, 'nobody is going to ruin my day'. It really works. It readjusts you so you can move on to the next task and stay in that good place in your head.

There is a solution to everything. The end result will not always turn out precisely as you planned as you may need to compromise a little depending on the circumstances. You are strong enough to deal with the fact that some plans need to be adjusted. Take a minute anytime you need. Don't rush into anything.

You don't have to deal with anything right now if it doesn't suit you. Take as much time as you need. Tell people you need to think about the situation and get back to them later. Only approach things when you are comfortable doing so. This takes the pressure off you and gives you the space you need to gather your thoughts. Be grateful that you can handle any situation and there is always help there if you need it. Do not be afraid to ask.

On a morning that you're finding it difficult to get out of bed, the days that you don't feel well, and motivation is low, try pressing the reset button and work on changing your thoughts, to more pleasant ones.

Start by turning on some music and use the tips above and try again. Take it nice and slow. Go one step at a time. You can turn things around and change your mood no matter how bad things get. Make the decision to take action. Pick whatever pleasant thing comes to mind. I sometimes get up just to have a cup of tea and a square of chocolate and before I know it, I am feeling better. I start cooking something or watering the plants. Take it gently. Listen to your body. This condition needs to be managed at a pace that you feel is suitable for you.

Ask yourself:
Who are the people in my life that make me feel happy, loved, understood?
What are my favourite things to do?
What is the best thing to ever happen to me?

You are bound to feel better after answering these questions. Plan something and do it. The results will give you something to look forward to. No matter how small, it doesn't matter. Just start moving towards it.

PRIORITISE YOUR PLANS AND
ADJUST ACCORDINGLY
BUT KEEP YOUR END GOAL FIXED.

DEALING WITH BEING OVERWHELMED

THE MORE YOU BREATHE, THE MORE CLEAR YOUR THOUGHTS BECOME AND THE MORE ARTICULATE YOU WILL BE.

What can you try when feeling overwhelmed? Everyone differs in their priorities. It depends on what is going on in your individual life at any one time.

You cannot base your priorities on other people's ideas or opinions. Just do what feels right for you. Nobody knows your body like you do. You need to have the motivation to do what you want to do. Set out your individual priorities. You need to feel strongly about what you are doing so that the motivation comes naturally.

You may need to take calculated risks – that is how we develop and grow. If you are overwhelmed by fear don't let it destroy all your plans.

IF THE PLAN DOESN'T WORK,
CHANGE IT.
KEEP THE GOAL.
EDIT THE PLAN
KEEP TWEAKING UNTIL IT WORKS
THE WAY YOU WANT IT TO.

Things to do:
Greet each day with a SMILE
Share
Be humble
Dream big
Respect and enjoy nature
Be nice
Do good deeds
Be yourself
Learn new things
Dance
Do not let fear put you off
Be flexible
Care
Enjoy life
Be present
Meditate
Be Kind
Forgive
Make collages with photos / cut outs
Stretch
Open and trust a little.

Don't feel guilty for doing what is best for you. Be fearless in the pursuit of what makes you happy. Do things that set your soul on fire. Giving up on your goals because of a setback or fear is like slashing your other 3 tyres because you got one flat one. Say YES to new adventures. Go for it! Do them at a pace that suits you.
Will it be easy? Probably not.
Will it be worth it? Absolutely! Yes!

Be around good energy, people you enjoy and who lift you up. Connect with people. Learn new things and grow. It's the best feeling in the world.

Life is a gift, and that gift is like glitter. You can throw a handful of it in the air, but when you try and clean it up, you will never get it all. Even long after the event, you will still find glitter in places to remind you of the good times, the special moments, the smiles you have had and will have in the future. Cherish the wonderful moments and hold onto them to carry you through the not so wonderful days. You are incredibly special in some peoples' eyes. Don't ever forget it!

"IF YOU CAN'T FLY...RUN
IF YOU CAN'T RUN...WALK
IF YOU CAN'T WALK...CRAWL
WHATEVER YOU DO KEEP MOVING FORWARD"
Martin Luther King

OPTIMISM

"A PESSIMIST SEES
THE DIFFICULTY
IN EVERY OPPORTUNITY
AN OPTIMIST SEES THE OPPORTUNITY
IN EVERY DIFFICULTY."
Winston Churchill

Optimism can turn a situation that looks negative or bleak into an opportunity or something to learn from. It can replace the draining thoughts of pessimism with something that will give you more positive energy and enthusiasm.

Optimism will help you to get over obstacles you face and to keep moving forward when you fall or stumble. Don't give up just because you have had some setbacks. Take it at your own pace and enjoy the process.

A good dose of optimism in your own life is essential and if you can introduce it in the lives of people around you, that is always a good thing. Sharing is caring. Optimism is contagious and you get a great feeling from helping others. If you're not an optimistic type of person, just start introducing a little of it daily into your life. If you persist enough you will notice the difference it makes and more will come. Remember, Rome wasn't built in a day.

Be enthusiastic. Here are some simple tips that can help you to get started.

- Be there for someone. Listen and lend an optimistic and grounded perspective to someone in your life who needs it. Helping others is unbelievably uplifting.
- You can do as much or as little as you're able for. At first, I find it best to just let the other person vent. Let them get their issue out into the open. Be there fully and listen. This might be enough. Just being there will help them to express emotional tension that has built up and get it out. If they get stuck in negative thinking or in making a mountain out of a molehill then it can be helpful to add your own perspective to ground them and to help shift their perspective on the situation. Try to make them see that if they zoom out, and distance themselves from the situation that things are not all that bad after all. They can see more clearly this way, and together the two of you might be able to find a solution, or a first step, that they can put into action. After taking the first step, they will begin to feel better and more in control of the situation.

- **Music**

Uplifting music is a great way to boost your mood and open new perspectives again. I use Bob Marley's song Three Little Birds. It never fails to put a smile on my face. It might do the same for you! You can do the same for people around you. Put on a positive song when you are with family and friends or send them an uplifting playlist.

- **Compliments**

Give people compliments and mean them! Be genuine and sincere. They can tell if you're faking it. Think about one thing that will make the other person smile, something good that they often take for granted about themselves. If you like it say it. Not everyone knows how to accept compliments. Don't be put off. Repeat the compliment if necessary. I usually say, "I'm telling you the truth".

- **Smile**

It always works. A smile makes you and the people around you instantly feel better. It works even when you don't feel that much like smiling. Try it and you'll see for yourself. If you are feeling a bit down, put a smile on your face, put your shoulders back, your chin up and see what happens to your mood.

- **Gratitude and appriciation**

Keep a gratitude journal and write down 3 things every day that you're grateful for. It can be family, friends, house, food, car, nature, sounds of the ocean, wind, children laughing etc.

Name 3 things you are grateful for right now. Be specific.

1.
2.
3.

- **Help others:**

Doing good does you good. Being busy with life can add a lot of tension and stress. People get overpowered and can't cope or even ask for help. If you see this, offer to help them. Volunteering is also good. I've found that the little volunteering I do for The Irish M.E. trust, which involves 2 hours a week, is enough for me. I set up a group in 2011 which gave me a purpose, helping to focus on others rather than myself. I find this very enjoyable. I had never done anything like this before, but I must say, it's definitely good for me. You could volunteer to call an old person and talk to them for 30 minutes a week. You could read for a visually impaired person or child. There are lots of things you can do. I must say it is extremely rewarding. Friendships are made along the way which is an added bonus.

Start helping someone in your life to wind down. Suggest going for a picnic, head off to your favourite spot and have a laugh together or perhaps you would like to go for a swim or a walk. You decide.
Sit together in silence and watch the clouds go by for a while. Chat and enjoy each other's company.

Cooking for a friend is a lovely thing to do or get a takeout and watch a movie and chill out together. Quality time with people near and dear to you is so enjoyable and it's what memories are made of.

The bonus is it will destress both of you.

- **Hugs**

Since Covid19 became a part of our lives, hugs have not been recommended but this will not always be the case. Never underestimate the power of a hug. They are simply the best and you don't need to say anything as the receiver will know that you care. Such a simple but loving gesture can mean a lot and lift someone's day.

Who are your favourite people to hug?
1.
2.
3.

A HUG CAN HELP TO MEND SOME OF THE BROKEN PIECES THAT LIFE CHIPS AWAY

Try this: Body wrap

I use this all the time and find it incredibly helpful for gathering myself before the day starts and grounding myself whenever I need it. Sometimes, I just do this because it feels so good. One day I was on the green outside the house with my neighbours' dogs, getting a bit of fresh air. When it came time to bring the dogs back in, they were having none of it! It was a beautiful day, and the sun was peeking out from behind the clouds, giving very pleasant heat that felt lovely on my face. The dogs were quite happy to frolic around the grass sniffing every blade that crossed their noses.

The larger of the two dogs decided to lay down and there was no moving him. He liked to roll and scratch on his back in the long grass and in fairness it looked very enjoyable, so I left him at it. I took this opportunity to tilt my face towards the sun and inhale a nice deep breath and then exhaled, releasing all the tension from my body, relaxing myself. Here in Ireland the sun is a rare thing as the weather is quite unpredictable. As I stood there, on the grass, I decided to do a Body Wrap.

Here's how you do it: Bring your attention to the top of your head and take a couple of deep breaths to let all the tension out of your body. When I breathe in I visualise all the negativity getting dragged up through my body and then I release it out on the exhale and relax my shoulders down and shake it all off. It is great for loosening tight muscles and freeing the body. My attention at this moment goes to my feet. I make a conscious effort at this stage to visualise roots going from my feet into the ground below to anchor me, so I feel grounded. Next, bring your attention back to the top of your head. Imagine you have a large silk cloth on top of your head. Now in a circular motion visualise the silk cloth wrapping itself around your head loosely like a bandage. Let it work its way down to your neck and shoulders. Feel them releasing tension. Move down to the chest and rib cage next, wrapping yourself all the way, keep going until you get to the waist and hips. At this stage you should be nicely relaxed, so keep going until you get to the knees and finally, you'll be at your ankles and feet. Now you're snug as a bug in a rug and well protected. Anything that comes at you during the day that is negative will bounce off your silk protection. You now have the power to choose what you let in. Be aware of this shield and remind yourself that nothing is going to get through only what you want to let in. I usually invite in love and kindness.

Finally take one last deep breath and anchor yourself into the ground with your imaginary roots. You are now in a great place to go about your day. Safely anchored to the ground.

Once you practice this a couple of times you can do it wherever you

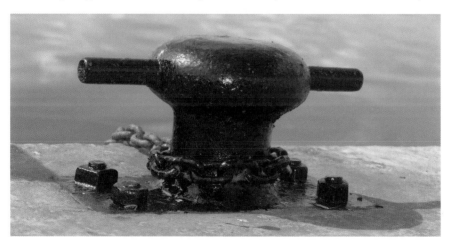

want. Like I said before, I was in the middle of the green with two small dogs and no one was the wiser to what I was doing while having my face tilted up enjoying the sun. I highly recommend you try this as it only takes a minute or two and you can do it as fast or slow as you wish. It is my protective blanket that I bring everywhere.

Earthing

Earthing is another excellent practice, and very healing for the body e.g. it reduces inflammation and increases antioxidants. Earthing is getting outside in your bare feet and walking in the grass. I believe that first thing in the morning is meant to be the best but anytime is good. The earth contains electrons that are absorbed through the feet and hugely beneficial to our wellbeing. This is stated in the book called *Earthing* by Clinton Ober. Clint is the CEO of Earth Fx Inc., a research and development company located in Palm Springs. He is the innovator behind the Grounding movement. This exercise grounds you and heals the body. For those of you interested in learning more about this, Clinton Ober's book is a good place to start. Dr. Stephen Sinatra M.D says it like getting a handful of antioxidants through your feet.

LIFE CAN BE A BUMPY ROAD
BUT WITH A DASH OF OPTIMISM
IT MAKES IT ALL THE BETTER.

What would you like to do more of in your life?
Be specific, for example, I like to watch wildlife. I would like to do more of it.
What are the areas in your life, that you want to grow and expand?
Name 3.
1.
2.
3.

What areas do you want to change for the better?

1.

2.

3.

What are your favourite things to do?

1.

2.

3.

If you were to write a letter to your 12-year-old self, what would your top 3 tips be:

1.

2.

3.

MADGE O'CALLAGHAN

Madge and I were introduced to each other by Declan from the Irish M.E. Trust in 2018. I joined in on an Amherst writing class once a month and we instantly clicked. When I told her that I was writing a book she offered to help. We had great fun and talked regularly regarding the book. Her help has been fantastic. I asked her to put a piece in the book as her knowledge is very extensive. Here is what she gave me.

Positive Deviance

I first came across the positive deviance approach at an international conference on women's mental health which took place in Dublin in 2016. The notion of positive deviance has fascinated me since.

Positive deviance is when a group or community of people have access to the same resources but use them differently with different degrees of success. It is a process that identifies how some people in a community, faced with the same constraints, and with access to no special or different resources to other members of the community, are able to overcome a particular problem. The concept was first identified in nutrition programmes. Some very poor families were discovered who had healthy, well-nourished children. When scientists studied these families, they realised that there were women in the community who were breaking with traditions and norms when feeding their families. These women were using their own initiative when it came to taking care of their children's diet. They fed them regularly and they included greens and small shrimps or crabs in their meals. These practices defied conventional wisdom which believed that these foods were dangerous or inappropriate for young children.

The concept of positive deviance also applies to many other problem situations. In trying to solve complex problems, leaders are inclined to turn to experts in the field, using a top down approach which does not always accomplish the solution to the problem. If we take the time to explore, there is usually someone in an organisation or a community who has already solved the particular problem we are stumped by. Someone, somewhere, has the answer to your problem or issue. These problem-solving people are living with the same resources and constraints as everyone else, yet they are able to harness their resources to achieve a better outcome for themselves and their families or community.

A good friend of mine was diagnosed with non-Hodgkin's lymphoma. She was in her twenties at the time. She had her spleen removed which left her vulnerable to infection. The hospital she attended sent her home and said that she may live for three months. She heard about a man in Scotland who had recovered from the same diagnosis. She wrote to him and he responded, telling her everything that he did to help him to recover from his cancer.

She began the process of getting well physically, spiritually, and mentally, based on the contents of the letter from a stranger. What had she to lose? She completely changed her diet. She juiced every day. She wasn't able to walk very far at the time and she set her mind on climbing Mount Errigal, a climb of almost 2,500 ft. She bought a pair of mountain boots and placed them on her bedside locker. Each morning they were the first things she would see, and each night before she went to sleep, they were the last things she would see.

At one point, she moved to a new house to be near the Bristol Cancer Centre to find out everything she could about recovery from her cancer. She became an expert in her own recovery. She once told me that she could tell the people in the centre who would recover from their curable cancers to those who wouldn't. The ones who would not recover were not able to make the adjustments necessary to get well. They often lacked the *confidence to make the changes needed in all the areas of their lives.*

She did get to climb Mount Errigal. She proudly displays her old boots now in the entrance hall of her home. They have a beautiful scene of Mount Errigal painted on them to remind her of her achievements. We spent her 60th birthday playing football on the beach at Kilkee. She is almost seventy now and an avid gardener, growing her own organic vegetables and taking her dog for long walks every day. She is one of the most upbeat people I have ever met. The most important thing the man had said to her in his letter was that she should choose to be happy and that she had to learn how to say no.

Now, I'm not claiming that everyone can recover from cancer – I wish that were true. Obviously, nowadays, some cancers are very treatable and have long lasting recovery rates. My friend's diagnosis was back in the 1970's. What I am saying is that there are those among us who will find solutions to their problems or issues that will give them the edge, the ability to solve whatever it is that is presented to them.

In dealing with fatigue, the experience and the expertise lies with those people who have found solutions that suit them. Finding a way of living with a condition such as M.E./CFS is unique to each individual. Happiness may not seem like a choice some days, but the more we practice being anything, the easier it becomes.

And as for saying no? Well, I think we can all learn how to say no assertively. Saying no is easy for babies and young children. It's quite often the first word a child will utter! As we grow, we pick up all sorts of negative messages about using the word "no". We may think it sounds mean or rude, or that we can't say no to someone because we may be letting them down.

For many years now I have been teaching people how to say "no" when they need to. It's not about saying no to everything. It's about choosing to say no to things that we really need to say no to so that we can genuinely say yes to things we want to do.

There are a couple of things to remember if you want to practice saying no.

Remember you have the right to say no.

When you are asked to do something, notice your immediate or gut reaction. What is it that your gut is telling you? Learn to listen to your gut. You will know straight away if it's a resounding Yes! We often resist the gut feeling if we are not sure what it is.

If you are not sure, ask for more information, e.g. How long will it take? How much will it cost?

If you have decided that you want to say no, be sure to say it clearly and directly. Many of us believe we are saying no when in fact we forget to use the little two letter word – no! Don't apologise – it diminishes the no when we start off by saying we're sorry. You might want to use self-disclosure e.g. "I really hate having to say this, but no, I don't want to meet you for coffee."

Repeat the "no" if necessary. "No, I'm not meeting you".

You might want to offer an alternative – but be genuine about this. Only offer an alternative if it's what you really want to do. "I'm happy to see you on Wednesday at the club and we can have a coffee there".

You might also want to enquire after the other person on the receiving end of the no.

Once you have been clear about saying no, move away physically or change the subject. Often, we find it difficult to say no and end up staying in the conversation with the other person and are persuaded to change our minds, so just stop the conversation or change it or move away.

Practice saying no in front of the mirror, or amongst trusted family or friends. One woman I knew always found herself buying things at the door from whoever came to sell to her. She ended up buying paintings she didn't want; food she didn't eat, even a carpet one time that she detested from the day it came into her house. She was sure she was saying no to the salespeople. When we role played the situation, she was indeed saying no to the sales people, but instead of being firm and saying no thank you and moving away to close her door, she was saying no and opening the door wider, giving the salespeople the opportunity to get her to change her mind.

When you practice saying no clearly and directly, you have a better chance of getting your message across to other people and leaving yourself open to the many opportunities to say yes.

COLM O'BRIEN

Colm and I crossed paths many years ago as our sons went to the same school. Over the years we met briefly on occasion, but it wasn't until years later that we became friends. Colm started doing the "Coffee at 11 Show" on zoom during Covid-19 and he invited me to be a guest. I was incredibly nervous at first, but he made me feel so comfortable that afterwards I was delighted that I participated. Colm is a complete gentleman and a wonderful character who has enriched my life.

Here are some words of wisdom from Colm.

The One Thing

"The Week is the Perfect Patch in the Fabric of Life". I love that phrase. I heard it first uttered by Stephen R Covey, author of The Seven Habits of Highly Effective People, on an audio program of the same name and instantly I got it. Think about it. Each week is exactly the same shape and size, seven days, each with 24 hours, 168 hours total, a beginning, middle and end, mornings, evenings, weekdays, a weekend – rinse and repeat.

Everything you do, everything I do, everything anyone does or has done at any point in history, or will at any point in the future, is done – happens - within a week, therefore it makes perfect sense to me at least that to become more effective in our lives, we must get better at making the weeks count. One way I have found to do that is to focus on making each week count and the easiest way to make the week count is to master The One Thing.

To begin to master The One Thing, I'd like to invite you to answer 4 questions.

1. On a piece of paper, or device, list the roles you play, in no particular order, just as they come to you, e.g. Mother, Father, Brother, Sister, Son, Daughter, Husband, Wife, Partner, Employee, Manager, Business Owner, Friend, Volunteer, Teacher, Coach, Board Member, etc. Try to think of as many as possible – how many different 'hats' do you wear in a week or a month?
Write now.

2. Now imagine your eightieth birthday. What date is it on? In what year? How many years is that from now? How do you feel about that? Is it so far away as to appear irrelevant? Is it so close as to feel scary? Regardless, I'd like you to answer a few questions about it:
• Who would you like to have in the room? Name 10
• What would you like the speaker to say about your life?
• What would you like them to say about your character and contribution?
• Think deeply. What achievements would you like them to remember? What impact would you have liked to have had on their lives?
Write now.

3. Now, revisit your roles. In the context of your Eightieth birthday, not in the context of where you are today, I'd like you to prioritize your roles. So, for example, based on the answers to your eightieth birthday question, which is the more important role, parent or volunteer, spouse, or business owner? There are no right or wrong answers by the way, just what's right for you, and nobody is judging.
Place the number 1 against the most important role you play today, as it relates to the picture you have formed for your eightieth birthday. Place the number 2 against the 2nd most important, no. 3 against the third and so on; you're getting the picture?
No need to split hairs on this exercise, no real need to debate which gets the no. 7 slot over the no. 8, or indeed no. 13 over no. 14! It's the top 3 to 6 we are looking for.

Write now.

4. Now. For each of your Top 3 roles, answer this question:
What One Thing, could you do in the next seven days (the next week)
that would have the biggest positive impact on your top role? Imagine
you could only do One Thing, but it would be significant, what would it
be? It could be to ring a friend, date your spouse, spend time with a child,
go for a walk alone, anything – what one thing could you do?
Now, commit. What One Thing WILL you do?
Write now.

You need to start living today with the picture of your own eightieth
birthday party clearly in your mind, because in that picture, you will
find your definition of true success. And if you practice The One Thing
each week, you can make it happen, one week at a time. Best wishes.

FINDING WAYS TO ADJUST TO THE NEW YOU

SLOW AND STEADY WINS THE RACE

Change takes time. It can all be a bit frightening and daunting at times. You may even experience fear and anxiety when life throws events at you. A few adjustments to the way you view things will make the world of difference. The changes you make will benefit you in the long run. You previously may have reacted to things in a less calm manner but now you don't bother as you know it will waste valuable energy. What you focus on at any one time will lead to the way you feel. Steer away from drama and confrontation. That is what you are reducing in your new chapter. You have turned over a new leaf. Leave the past behind you and face the future with optimism. There is lots of good research about M.E./CFS going on around the world that will benefit us.

The first thing to do is to breathe and relax. There is no rush. When someone asked you to do something in the past you might have been stressed out and got flustered and just said yes without thinking. The new you will pause and think about things for a moment and decide, "Do I really want to do this?" or "can I do this?" if you don't want to answer straight away, that's perfectly alright. It's your rules now, and your pace.

The new you will deal with all that life throws at you in a calmer fashion.

Remember:
• Don't miss out on something wonderful that could be around the corner.
• Falling is an accident. Staying down is a choice.
• Being happy never goes out of style.
• Don't let anyone steal your smile.
• Don't let anyone ruin your day.
• Don't complain about things you are not willing to change. Either do it or set it free.

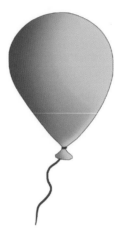

Cut the balloon
Whenever I have a concern or I'm fretting about something and can't get it out of my mind, I try this. I imagine I have a balloon in my hand and a piece of string. I blow up the balloon and fill it with all the thoughts I want to get rid of. Once I am content that I have everything in there I tie it up with the piece of string and let it fly in the air while still holding onto it. Once I'm happy that it's time to let go, I take an imaginary scissors out of my pocket and cut the string. I visualise the balloon flying off into the sky watching as it lifts higher and higher. Then I say good-bye to my troubles and ask the universe to take care of them. This works really well and lightens my mood instantly.

I heard a lovely story about balloons that I would love to share with you. It goes like this:

A teacher brought balloons to school. One was given to every child. Each child had to write their name on the balloon they were given and then place it in the hallway outside the room. The teacher then mixed up all the balloons. The children were requested to find their own balloon. Despite a hectic search, no one found their balloon. They were then asked by the teacher to pick the balloon nearest to them and hand it to the person beside them. They were all happy now as they each had a balloon. The teacher explained to them all that the balloons are like happiness. We will never find it if everyone is looking for their own. Whereas if we care about other people's happiness, we will find ours too.

I love this story as it is so true. Focussing on others is such a joy.

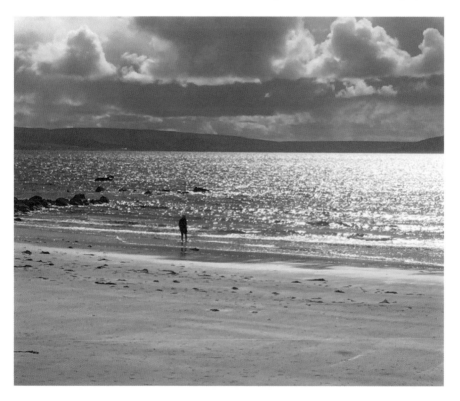

FREEDOM

Be aware of the following areas and work on them.

Worrying
Worrying is like walking around with an umbrella waiting for it to rain, pointless! Yes? When you notice yourself worrying over something you have no control over or that might never happen, flip it quickly by focussing on benefits you can get from whatever you are doing. Worrying gets you nowhere and is unbelievably bad for your health.

Courage
Courage doesn't mean you don't get afraid. It means you're not going to let fear stop you from getting the results you are after. Stop being afraid of what could go wrong and think of what will go right. You will be able to deal with things as they arise and know that you can handle them. Don't let anyone rent space in your head unless they are good to you. In other words, don't rehash old conversations that were unpleasant. Overthinking is soul destroying. Be aware of your thoughts and stop them from driving you crazy. Allow the good in and the bad out.

Keep going, you will get there. Things will get better. Let no one discourage you. You don't need a fan club to achieve your goals. Be your own motivator. It is good to fall asleep with a dream and wake up with a purpose. Write down in your diary something you want to do the following day. This will help you to get motivated.

BE IN THE MOMENT
LISTEN MORE, TALK LESS.
CONSERVE YOUR ENERGY

Conserving energy
Truly and fully listening in conversations, has been one of my biggest challenges to date. Anyone who knows me, knows I'm a talker and I get excited about things and get caught up in the moment. I love life and wasting energy on chatting to everyone is what I did for years.

I started going to a specialist to manage my M.E./CFS better and she gave me some tips.

- You don't have to talk to everyone.
- Sit back and take in the room. Let people come to you.
- If there is someone you would particularly like to talk to, get up every now and again and head over to them.
- Limit your time at any party e.g. three hours at most. There will be the odd occasion where you have to stay longer but mostly limit it so you're not getting burned out.
- Take it easy for a couple of days after if you notice fatigue. One of my warning signs is when my voice gets deeper. Then I know I have to slow down and take extra rest.
- Learn to recognise your own warning signs and take action straight away.

Listening

In the last few years, I have made an effort to become a better listener. I can't say I do it well in every conversation, but I believe I have improved a lot.

Listening is a win/win

I find that if I listen better, I enjoy other people's company more. I focus on understanding people and taking in what they are saying. This deepens relationships and makes true and lasting connections. One of the best ways to remember something, and stay in listening mode, is to pretend that you are going to tell what you learnt to someone else. Then you'll be more alert to what is said in the conversation. Everything just simply seems to stick better in my experience. You're not going to tell anyone as it's a private conversation with a friend but just use the tactic to help you stay tuned in and listen. By using this technique you'll also start asking more follow-up questions naturally, because you'll become more interested and you want to understand more deeply.

This also makes the person that is talking to you, feel more understood and appreciated and so your conversation and relationship will be better.

LIFE & CHALLENGES

Do any of you find that when you start cleaning your room you find things you forgot about? And then start getting distracted by them and never get the job done?
Do I hear a yes?

Challenges are what make life interesting and overcoming them is what makes life meaningful.

Awareness is vital. Be interested in what you are dealing with. Have consideration and care about things around you.

Take action
Choose your friends wisely. Be with those that lift you up and make you feel better about yourself. Always find things you love to do and that make you feel happy. Make a list. There are always people that want to bring you down and push your buttons. Don't waste your time and energy on these people. It will do you no good. Life is too short. Draw a line and don't bother arguing. Set your boundaries.

STRONG WOMEN DON'T HAVE ATTITUDES.
WE HAVE PRIORITIES AND BOUNDARIES.
CHALLENGES MAKE US STRONGER

Challenge yourself to stop complaining.
Could you do it for a week?
Or even a couple of days?
Are you up for it?

One of the greatest challenges we face is to not fear other's opinion of us. It takes a lot of strength to stand tall and say what you need to say calmly and freely. When I want to feel strong, I visualise being the lion. I see myself standing tall on the edge of the mountain and looking out over the valley. The sense of freedom I get when I stand there with not a care in the world, is so liberating. I say to myself what it is I need to say. I shout if I need to or roar like a lion and feel the release.

There is a lot of misunderstanding about M.E./CFS. It is important to release the frustration that this misunderstanding causes in you. The challenges we face are real! It astounds me how the World Health Organisation (WHO) can recognise this illness and some doctors don't. In some countries people with M.E./CFS have tolerated dubious treatment of their condition. Governments apologised and vowed to look after them and accepted that this condition seriously affects the body. M.E./CFS is a neurological condition and this has been proven. Anyone who does not understand that at this stage needs to educate themselves. It is not acceptable for one person to give another a hard time over having M.E./CFS.

Many of us with M.E./CFS find it difficult to find a doctor who understands this condition. Not every doctor will know everything. I have been to many. My GP is super but there have been times when he has had to refer me to other specialists e.g. neurological specialist for migraines, respiratory specialists for asthma. When dealing with anyone stay strong, calm, and confident. Express what you need to say. It might take being persistent and visiting a few different doctors. This is disappointing as we do not have the energy to waste. Some doctors are dismissive and condescending. This is not acceptable. If this happens to you walk away and get someone who treats you with the respect you deserve!

I have had my fair share of negative experiences with doctors. One experience stands out clearly. A specialist sat in front of me and told me that what I was describing was not possible. The experience was very real for me. I was home alone and not able to breathe. At the time I had chronic asthma and had very severe blockages of my windpipe/ oesophagus with phlegm which caused immense difficulty in breathing. On this particular day, I really got a fright as I could not clear the phlegm. Eventually, with great difficulty, I cleared my airway and was able to breathe again. I got an awful fright and that's why I had gone to the specialist. She didn't believe me, which was shocking! She said that what I was saying was not possible! She agreed to do some tests, but the problem was she did not believe or understand what had happened to me. She had not come across this before and concluded it was impossible. Others may not have been as lucky as I was. People can die from asthma. If they are dead, they can't tell you what happened! I was lucky to have survived.

In the end she told me it was more than likely asthma and that I had to continue managing it as I had been. End of story!

I realised at that stage I needed to make some serious decisions. I definitely didn't want to experience what I had before. I had to do something different. I bought a nebuliser for my home. This helped to keep the airways open. The next thing I did was to cut back dairy as it is mucus forming and mucus was what caused the problem in the first place. This helped so much that I cut it out altogether. I have been off dairy now over 3 years and the difference to the amount of medication I take for asthma has also reduced. I'm not the only one with asthma who has chosen to give up dairy and noticed a huge difference. One lady I met said her mother was a doctor and wasn't in favour of her giving up dairy. When she saw the results her daughter had, it converted her. Now the whole family has made the switch.

I also made sure that when I get an infection in my chest that from day one, I have my nebuliser at hand. I use steam every day, 3 times a day and vapour rub on my chest, back and the soles of my feet at night. This helps a lot along with steroids and strong antibiotics.

The changes I made to my diet and management of my asthma, have helped enormously with the reduction of phlegm, so much so I haven't had a scare like that again. The point I am making here is that you will be challenged and not believed but whatever happens, your experiences are real.

Talk to your doctor about food allergy testing. There is a difference between food allergy and sensitivity. Allergies are not good and need to be addressed. If I had taken a food allergy test earlier, I would have discovered dairy as one allergen for me.

No doctor or specialist suggested giving up dairy or getting allergy testing which is surprising to me.

Find ways that help you adjust to your new reality. Touch off one area at a time. I suffered from migraines for fifteen years and nobody helped me. Finally, I was told about an acupuncturist, Dheai Isaaid, who is a General Oriental Practitioner and is fantastic. Dheai owns the East West Clinic. It took a year of treatment but in the end my migraines reduced by 95%.

Opinions

Everyone has an opinion, and they are entitled to it. You have the power to agree to differ. If you have a particular situation that you want to change, you can't change other people's opinion, but you can change how your reaction is to that opinion. You don't have to disagree or react. Try pausing before you react or speak as this gives you time to gather your thoughts. Sometimes you may choose not to speak at all. Think about it. Does it really matter what they think? Most of the time it doesn't. If you do choose to speak, take your time, and get to the point quickly.

Don't get too upset if someone has a different opinion to you. Having M.E./CFS can result in people around you having opinions regarding the illness that are sometimes unpleasant. This is difficult. Know that you have done nothing wrong. That is just their perspective on things.

Take a good look at yourself and ask yourself:
What do I need to do to make the best of this situation? Then just relax and take it all in your stride.

If you must approach somebody about a situation you don't like, try the following:

- Be prepared before you have the conversation and have a plan.
- Get to the point quickly.
- Ask for their help if necessary, to improve the situation.
- Don't be scared to speak up and say what it is you need to say.
- If people in your life are insensitive, draw a line in the sand regarding what you will tolerate.

Stop them from eroding your confidence.

- Don't be in ANY SITUATION that you're unhappy with.
- You can make changes to your life and design the life you want with the people you want in it.
- Don't be immobilised by fear. It's ok to have an opinion.
- Stand up and be strong. Follow your gut and stop behaviour you don't want or like. Life is too short. It's time to be happy and content.
- Don't let people put you on a guilt trip. It's ok to say NO. I realise it can be very difficult but it's a necessity for us to care for ourselves. Our limitations are real and not everybody will see that. We need to do what we can and say NO to what we can't. People may not like it, that's too bad. Stick to your guns and do what you feel you can handle.
- Don't be a victim. Do something about the situation, so that you are comfortable and content.

You can change any situation. Just pause and breathe and get to the point. Stay grounded. You are in charge.

Example: Someone is being disrespectful to you. It may be a child or an adult. This needs to be stopped. You say what you don't like, and you move on. You may have to address it again as people take time to change their ways. You address the situation again when it arises. Eventually, they will see you don't tolerate this kind of behaviour.

The past is the past. Today is a new day and you need to choose to be respected and happy in your life. Choose to move on and be brave.

You will get stronger! Don't mind what you used to be. This is the new you. Keep your chin up and move on.

Ask yourself:
"What do I want?" "How am I going to get it?"

A few things to try when dealing with difficult people.

If somebody insults you e.g. you look really tired today, say "thanks for that, it really makes me feel better". This will hand it back to them, so you don't accept it and let it in. Remember your body wrap exercise on page 146.

When someone insults you in a very mean way ask them "Can you repeat that slowly?" Chances are they won't. You have now brought attention to the situation and others might hear and they don't want that.

If that doesn't work and they do repeat it ask them "Are you trying to hurt my feelings? If so, you're wasting your time". And smile.

Insults only work if you let them in and take them personally. It ends up like a game of tennis. You can't play tennis if your opponent doesn't return your serve.

THERE IS NO SUCH THING AS FAILURE.
YOU ALWAYS ACHIEVE SOMETHING
WHEN YOU TAKE ACTION.

CELEBRATE

IN DEFEAT AND SUCCESS
CELEBRATE!

Celebrating is especially important as you feel so much better after it. Every step of the way is an achievement. If you succeed, great. If you don't, move on. You have learnt something valuable from the experience. You gave it a shot and you deserve a WELL DONE for moving beyond your comfort zone.

Raise your hand in the air. Bring it down behind your back and give yourself a pat on the back.

Have an open mind. Let the ideas flow. If you were doing a drawing you might make many attempts before you get the desired finish. You'll change direction while you're doing it. New ideas might pop into your head. It might take longer than you expected. You'll feel it when it's right. You'll know it.

If the seeds of doubt come, blow them away. You never know what's around the corner. Keep learning and growing. Listen and be open to the possibilities, and act on them.

Remember:
- Don't make excuses that will result in you doing nothing. You can

talk yourself out of anything.
- Choose wisely what you want and go for it.
- Don't complain. If you don't like something, change it.
- Variety is the spice of life.
- Challenge yourself. Try something new.

Suggestions:
- Cook something new.
- Listen to a new Podcast
- Meditate for 5 minutes a day.
- Plant a new flower in your garden and watch it grow and flourish.
- Make a new friend

It's up to you to decide. If you try new things, you'll know what feels good then you can build on that. Otherwise move on to the next thing on your list to try.

YOU ARE HERE. YOU ARE BREATHING AND YOU HAVE
MORE TO GIVE. LIFE IS ABOUT GROWING.
LOOK AROUND YOU.

HOW TO OVERCOME PERFECTIONISM

STRATEGIES FOR MAKING
A BETTER LIFE

Perfectionism can lead to tearing your hair out every time things don't turn out the way you want or how you pictured. Frustration gets on top of you. Perfection is extremely hard to achieve. Everyone's idea of perfection is different so to try and be perfect is unrealistic. If we stop trying to be perfect, and acknowledge that we are human, this will help us be more content.

Perfection paralyses us and puts massive pressure on people. If you're doing a task and you are uptight about getting it done perfectly, it may prevent you from doing it well. Relax.

We all want to make things better, don't we? Being a perfectionist at your job or in your life slows everything down. Open your mind and try things out. Try looking at all the possibilities. You can keep your target the same, just be open minded and not so rigid.

This will not affect your ability to do a good job. In fact, it will improve your outcome. Not only will you get the job done, the people around you, will be far happier and content. Working together is the key. Be flexible and listen to other opinions. Unrealistic expectations for everything being perfect isn't the answer. It causes frustration, anger and will burn up a lot of your energy.

We can regroup at any stage and change the plan and move on. We can be the moving part. Reality will not budge, but our expectations can. We will still get to the desired destination. Mistakes will happen - that's life - they can be fixed. You simply adjust and move on.

There will always be wrinkles to be ironed out so be flexible. Next time around we will be more effective. This is how we learn and grow. So instead of concluding: "That didn't work at all!" we could think, "That didn't work yet," or, "Some of that worked, and some of it didn't. What do I need? What is my next step?" Progress can be slow, and attempts can be many, but if you get there in the end that is all that matters. Go back to the drawing board as many times as needed. Keep adjusting until it all fits. It will all lead us to be a better, stronger person in the end.

So, learn to accept the bumps in the road and roll with the punches. Work through and enjoy your successes and achievements. You might not succeed in the way you imagined right away but hanging in through the process is how you strive for progress over time.

When we embark on a new project instead of falling into the trap of perfectionism, we can do ourselves a favour and decide to take things as they come.

Ask yourself:
What is working for me now?
What am I enjoying?
"Why isn't this working? Can I do something differently?"

Just keep moving forward to what is next. Each step is crucial so finish one and move onto the next. This is what I was told when doing a project or when I was working in a shoe shop while in school. The manager told me "one customer at a time, do not look at the big line of people to be served. Just deal with what's in front of you. That way you don't panic and get afraid and overwhelmed"

Sit back and take a good look at the whole thing. Separate the wood from the trees. Divide it all up based on importance. Some parts need extra effort. Enjoy the getting there as much as being there at the end.

Enjoy what you're doing, discipline yourself to have a cut-off point. You can come back to it again later. Whether you're preparing for a child's birthday party, repainting a room, or preparing for a speech, we're more likely to do better when we can find the enjoyment or purpose in what we are doing. When we are tense, it does us no good, and we cannot think straight, and it narrows our field of vision. When we are enjoying what we do our brains work so much better and our enthusiasm helps us be more creative. The people around us are a great deal happier also.

What causes despair and convinces us we should abandon a task, or at least procrastinate about working on it, is finding one thing not going well. We then can conclude that the whole thing is not working. When this happens, just breathe and after a minute or two adjust the things that are not working and move on.

Take it easy on yourself. Not everything is urgent. Try to take a breather. Your life will carry on if you leave the plates in the sink. The floor can wait to be washed. It's not going anywhere. The boss will not fire you if you make a mistake. Not everything can be of maximum importance in your life. Sure, we all have priorities and that's perfectly fine. Try being kinder to yourself and a little more flexible.

Name 3 areas where you can take a softer approach. It can be with people or things. Gently does it.
1.
2.
3.

Here are a few ideas:
• Speak kinder to the people around you. I realise people can drive you crazy and sometimes you just want to lash out at them. Being blunt is not always the way to go. You will regret the words said afterwards.
• Try driving without cursing everyone who does something silly on the road.
These simple acts will conserve energy you can put to better use later.

Remember:
- Take a deep breath and look at what you did wrong. See what you can do to fix it.
- Try connecting with others rather than criticising them. Compliments are far more effective than putting others down.
- Express your gratitude. A simple please and thank you goes a long way.
- Send someone a nice text.
- See people for who they are. We are all different and that is a good thing. Respect people's ways and realise we all have quirks and opinions.

Can you try for one week to see the good in others?

The grass is not always greener on the other side. We all have issues in our lives. We may not talk about them, but they are there. Everything may look rosy on the outside. People have ways of hiding behind masks. Just because somebody is beautiful and well-dressed doesn't mean they are happy. That's the outside and we cannot see what's going on inside. I feel that a lot of us, me included, try to pretend we don't have M.E./CFS as there is still a lot of stigma attached to it. We don't want people treating us differently or feeling sorry for us.

It's like the beautiful swan, elegant and graceful gliding through the water but underneath the feet are paddling furiously.

We don't know what goes on behind closed doors. Be kind and find a way to enjoy other people's company. We are not in a competition. Try not to begrudge others or put yourself down for not having what they have. This will lead to you being very unhappy.

We can improve the quality of our lives by adjusting the way we feel and the way we think. Let's free ourselves from striving for perfection. If at first you don't succeed, try again and learn lots along the way. None of us knows it all so make some mistakes. It's perfectly normal.

Sarah Warde

Sarah Warde

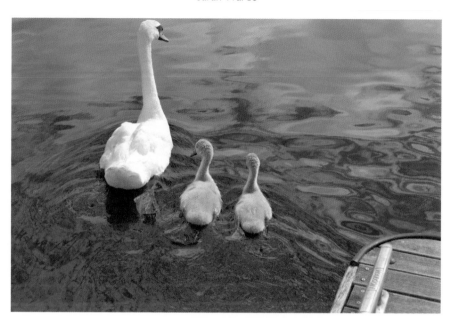

GOALS v POSSIBILITIES

ENJOY THE ENDLESS POSSIBILITIES, EVERYDAY BRINGS.

Don't wait until you've reached your goal to be proud of yourself. Be proud of every step you take towards reaching that goal.

When you get an idea write it down immediately!

Then:
Plan, prioritise, commit, and take action. Nothing will ever happen until you make a move in the right direction and start working on it.
Be patient. Don't rush in and do it all at once. You will run out of steam.
Try the fifteen-minute rule.
Set the alarm for fifteen minutes and then stop and revisit the task the following day and the day after that.
This will save energy and you won't end up over-exerting yourself.
Persistence is essential. How often have we heard "Patience is a virtue?"
Breathe and gather your thoughts.
Nice and steady does it.

Tips:
- Focus on the destination, not the journey.
- Set realistic amounts of time to complete goals so as not to be under pressure and cause anxiety.
- Be realistic and consider any factors that may be outside your control.
- Goals can be adjusted and rewritten, they are not set in stone. Things happen.

In life we need to seek pleasure, happiness, freedom, and excitement. By consciously seeking them you will bring more of them into your life. That's what we are aiming for.

Bring in simple luxuries into your daily life

Have a bubble bath, watch a nice movie, have a cup of tea with a good friend. Enjoy the nature and beauty around you. Be content by yourself and mix with others so you can grow, learn, and build meaningful connection.

Talk to interesting people. Mix with all sorts so you become aware of different opinions attitudes and behaviours. Also, you will discover what makes people tick and what stories they have. My husband and I met a lovely couple who were travelling through Ireland, we were in a pub in Liscannor at the time. We just sat back and listened to their stories, and they did the same. Good times. It was great fun and we learnt lots about where they came from and their travels.

A few years back I fractured my ankle and ended up sitting in a waiting room for an hour before I got seen. Beside me was a large man, about 6'5" and about 18 stone, with lots of tattoos. Normally, as I am 5'3" I might have been intimidated by such a character, only because I didn't know him. We ended up chatting to each other and had the most interesting conversation. He was a biker and had travelled to some fabulous places. He really was a gentle giant. I told him how glad I was to have met him and wished him all the best as he went in to his appointment. He had fallen off his bike and broken his arm. I was later telling my husband about my encounter and how we can't judge a book by its cover. Now I'm not saying to go and talk to everybody, take a calculated move when it feels right and strike up a conversation. It makes life more interesting.

My dad used to tell me to talk to everyone as you will learn something from every conversation you have. Great advice from a great man.

Your goal is to feel good and be happy.
Bring your attention to the inside of your body. Pick a spot. I usually pick the tummy area. Become aware of your feelings and become familiar with them. Get used to them and turning them around. You are in charge of your feelings.
Remember the visualisation exercise earlier in this book regarding your mood. See page 35.
Be enthusiastic. Make a plan and go for it. Don't overthink it.
Trust in yourself that you are capable of getting a pleasant result

Divide life into sections like a pizza and make lists:
Example:
- Family
- Relationships
- Friends
- Happiness
- Health
- Hobbies
- Education
- Travel

You cut the pizza slice to a size that suits you, depending on your priorities e.g. family may be more important to you than education. You decide.
Treat yourself to a vision / possibilities board. Fill it up with what you dream of. Have some fun. When you look at your board it will reflect visually what your inner wishes are. Put up that picture of the kitchen you'd love, the car you want, the holiday you dream of etc.

Next thing, decide how and what you're going to do about getting it. Just by looking at your board every day and enjoying it will attract what you want into your life. You can have more than one board. Put one in your kitchen and one in your bathroom or study. This way when you are reading or meditating you can look at the board and visualise yourself having what you see on it. This will bring a smile to your face and a good feeling in your heart.

Everything is possible

DO NOT DISMISS anything! Look into ALL the possibilities and get all the details.

Then decide what your plan of action is. Remember, you don't have to commit to anything until you have all the information. Then sleep on it. If you still feel it's a good idea, then go for it and enjoy.

Enjoy meeting your goals. When I was writing this book, I never thought in my wildest dreams I would do anything like this, but as I took it on, bit by bit it came together. I wrote most of it from my bed. My husband used to tease me about finding pens in the bed. When I asked him to print out the book one day, he was shocked at what he saw. He never teased me again.

Set your goal and see what it is you want to achieve. Look at the end result and work back from there, i.e. lose weight, get organised, etc.

Start with small achievable goals and work your way up. This builds confidence.

Things will always throw you off course as nothing is certain in life but when you get comfortable with uncertainty, infinite possibilities open up to you and your life will change dramatically.

This will mean fear is no longer a dominant factor in your life and is not preventing you from achieving your goals and possibilities. You will start to enjoy the excitement of it all and know that you are going to be just fine because you are able to handle any situations. You will feel more energetic and alert and ideas will start flowing again.

Your inner voice:

Watch your inner voice as it can be extremely negative. Before I worked on my inner voice, I was making life difficult for myself. I was awfully hard on myself, constantly thinking I was not good enough and feeling very insecure.

I put on a good exterior act and you wouldn't have guessed it. Inside was a whole different ball game.

Thought management

Once I became aware of thought management in my life things started to change. Be aware of your thoughts and manage them – changing the negative to positive. Flip it like a pancake. Having a negative inner voice can bring you down faster than the Titanic if it goes unchecked.

Unhappy people can have terribly negative thoughts and put themselves down a lot. They will spread that in your direction if you're not careful. So, steer clear and keep them at a distance or minimise the time you spend with them.

Your inner critic may be one of your biggest obstacles standing in your way to getting the happiness you wish.

If you make a mistake or fail, that's okay. This will build your character. Just give it another go. If someone criticises you, then your inner voice can become louder and louder and drag you down and keep you from doing what you wish to do. Your motivation will go out the window. Be aware of how your thoughts are flowing and change the direction when needed as quickly as possible. If they are negative, they can fill your head with all kinds of crazy things e.g. you're not good enough, not pretty enough, not bright enough etc. Stop and breathe and change direction. A wonderful lady called Moira Geary who was the first guest into our Limerick group, told me once "Erase and delete". This works really well. Now when I think bad thoughts that bring me uneasy feelings, I erase and delete. When I move on it's in a different more uplifting direction.

Being able to turn the inner critic around or quieten it as soon as it pops up is a particularly useful skill.

Here are two simple steps to help you

1. Say STOP

In your mind tell yourself to STOP! as soon as you become aware of what you're doing. When your critic pipes up knock it on the head.

My other favourite is to say "No! No! I am not going there!"

This will disrupt your train of thought before it gets bigger and more powerful.

2. Remind yourself what these negative thoughts will lead to, if you continue to think like this.

After you have said stop, remind yourself of the cost to your self-esteem if you continue. As someone said to me. "It's just too expensive to do that, so don't."

The cost to your mind, body and wellbeing is way too high. Who wants to be in an unpleasant situation where you are miserable? No-body!

Remind yourself how the inner critic has shaped your life so far.

See how the cost of letting your thoughts roam free for another year will affect you. This doesn't just affect you but the people around you as well.

This reminder makes it a lot easier to say no and to let go of such destructive thoughts. Replace them with ones that benefit you and the world around you a lot more.

You will find that motivating and kind thoughts when you have a setback or hit a bump in the road will be hugely beneficial.

THE SECRET TO HAPPINESS IS LETTING EVERY
SITUATION BE WHAT IT IS, INSTEAD OF
WHAT YOU THINK IT SHOULD BE.

Name 3 things you do that take you to your happy place

1.

2.

3.

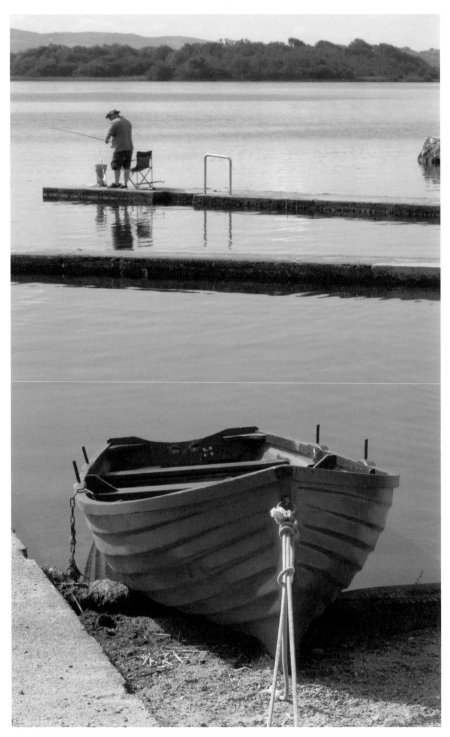

STRESS

A lot of stress can build up not only for ourselves but for others around us. Having a serious health condition that limits your ability to carry out regular daily activities like others is incredibly stressful. For me, if someone asks me to go somewhere with them, I must make sure that I will be able to keep up. If there is a lot of walking involved, then that's a no no for me. If you find yourself in this position, think of ways around your obstacles. Do the people you're going with understand your condition and your limitations? Are they flexible, kind and understanding? The last thing you need is someone to give you a hard time because you can't keep up.

Let's take a look at those who are in a relationship and the stresses involved. De-stressing is particularly important in a relationship and needs to be regularly addressed. Stress impacts our nearest and dearest more than we realise. It is exceedingly difficult to watch your loved ones not be able to live the life they used to live and to give up on their careers, activities, and dreams. Everything that was completely normal now has obstacles attached.

Pacing and planning are the new norm.
Stress has become part of our lives and there is no way to avoid it but there are ways to control it. We need to do something about stress

because ignoring it is not the solution. It only makes it worse. Stress is also contagious as you can feel the vibes from the other person and you automatically tense up. You become afraid that you will say or do the wrong thing and set the other person off.

The first thing to do is to try and open up about it. Communication is the key to it all. Now that's not always easy but be patient and kind about it and take it slow. Nobody is at fault. Remember it's just life. There is no room for judgement. Just listen and try to understand.

Examples of short-term stress is fighting, being disconnected from each other, sadness, frustration, etc. On the other hand, you have long term stress that can turn into bad health, e.g. depression.

The next thing to do after you have acknowledged and talked about your stress is to figure out ways to help each other overcome it together. One thing is to know your partner's behaviour and be aware when it's off. Is he/she angry, moody, argumentative, teary, withdrawn, hyper, or overly excited? Keep an eye out for an increase in alcohol, food, and drug consumption.

It is especially important to listen to each other without judgement. Stay calm as there is a solution to your challenges. You must be united and work through them together. The sun will shine again as this too shall pass.

Do things together like walks, read, cook, star gaze, picnics etc. These are great to help you relax and open up. I usually go to the beach as I find the sea is very therapeutic and calming. Go for a little walk and find a nice spot to sit and chat. Relax and listen to the ocean and the birds. Enjoy your surroundings. Bring a nice picnic with some of your favourite treats included. Chill out and have a laugh together. Don't rush into the subject. Then when the time is right, approach the topic gently.

Forming habits

I have found over the past few years, that If I really try to stick with one thing at a time, it reduces stress, and everything becomes easier and easier as time goes by.

You can pick whatever you wish and just stick with it. Once you feel it has become a habit and you don't have to try so hard, as it will becomes second nature, move onto the next area you wish to change. If you do too much at any stage, you will become overwhelmed and annoyed. You will end up getting slapped back to square one. I tried fighting this condition for years. Looking back, it did more harm than good. When I did not listen to my body and what it was telling me, I ended up exhausted and unable to do anything.

Name 3 habits you want to change.

1

2.

3.

    Habits are something we all have, and they are possible to change if needed. We have good ones and not so good ones that don't help us at all.

    The first thing we need to do is to be aware of which habits we wish to change and then go about adjusting them slowly. It takes about six weeks to alter behaviour and to form new habits.

Be gentle with yourself. Enjoy what you are doing, knowing that this is for you. You will know what you are able for. Don't push too hard as this will lead to stress.

RELAXATION AND THE IMPORTANCE OF IT

YOU HAVE ENOUGH
YOU DO ENOUGH
YOU ARE ENOUGH
SO RELAX

Here is something I like to do as it helps me relax and ground myself. You can do it anywhere. For this example, I am going to take you to the beach. My husband and I love listening to the sound of the ocean.

As we stand on the edge of the water, we do the following:
Clear our minds and take a deep breath in. We repeat this 3 times.
Using all our senses one at a time, we name
5 things we can see
4 things we can hear
3 things we can feel
2 things we can smell
1 thing we can taste
This is a fantastic thing to do and it clears the head of all the other thoughts and leaves you feeling so much better.

Remember:
- Do one thing at a time and do it slowly and mindfully.

- Connect deeply with people and nature.
- Meditate frequently.
- Appreciate silence.
- Expect nothing.
- Be grateful for everything.
- Observe without judgement.
- Consume less and create more.
- Let go of your past, all the fears and anxieties.
- Have a purpose in your life.
- Listen to others, understand, and care.
- Know you can't fix everything, but you can make it better.
- Be patient with yourself and others.
- Love with all your heart.
- Don't complicate things, keep it simple and go step by step until you get where you wish to go.

There is a lot to be said for just sitting and observing what is around you at any given time. My favourite spot to do this is by the sea, but you can do it anywhere you like.

Just take a few minutes out of your day and watch and breathe. I was just looking out the window and I spotted a robin. He looked like he hadn't a care in the world as he hopped from branch to branch. Then he flew away, and it felt so freeing. I wished for a minute I could be that robin, even for a day. Just to see how it felt. Maybe in my next life.

Recently I was on a trip to Doolin, in Clare. I went down by the rocks and just sat there taking it all in. I watched the birds gliding in the currents in the wind and I watched on so enviously as it looked so peaceful. In the background you could see the vast ocean in its magnificence. The sun was reflecting on the sea below. The sparkles were bouncing around. What a picture it made! People came and went as I sat there, and each were amazed by the sheer beauty of it all. I sat listening to the waves crashing off the rocks with a big smile of contentment across my face. It was so tranquil that I closed my eyes and just listened and took a great big deep breath in so I could set my body completely free. I gave into the wonderful peaceful feeling that washed over me. Everything else just dissolved and I was left in a state of deep relaxation that I wished I never had to leave. The magic of the senses come into play, i.e. smell, touch, sight, hearing, and taste.

As I sat there, I could feel the warm breeze blow past me and the taste of the salt as it landed on my mouth. I can smell the seaweed wafting by my nose. I started to crave a good old bag of chips with lots of salt and vinegar. The waves rolling in were beautiful and the sound was hypnotic. It was truly amazing. I had to leave this setting to go back to reality, but I took my time and enjoyed every minute of the spectacular surroundings. I made my way back to Lahinch for the chips and they were delicious and well worth the wait.

Getting away from the hustle and bustle of everyday life is very necessary and I realise you may not be able to go to the sea every day unless you're lucky enough to live there. The good news is you don't have to. We are all gifted with a wonderful imagination. You can visualise anything you want, and your brain can't tell the difference. So, if you are feeling overwhelmed during your day just take a time out. It can be anything from five to fifteen minutes. You decide. Go to your magical place and notice the difference you feel afterwards. I find I can even smell the ocean. The mind is truly magical, and this is a great advantage to have.

Try this:

When I was younger, I used to love skimming stones on the ocean surface. My friends and I would have bets on who'd achieve the most skips of the stone on the water until the final plonk and it sank to the bottom. I lost a lot and would have to give up some of my sweets, but it was worth it for the laughs we had.

Nowadays when I return to beaches, I take off my shoes and feel the sand between my toes. I walk towards the shoreline and search for the perfect stone. A smile comes to my face as I get myself ready and just before I release the stone, I attach a thought to it. One I no longer want. I send the thought flying off with the stone over the surface of the water where it eventually sinks down to the ocean bed. There it stays. Finally, I take a big deep breath and let it all go and it feels wonderful.

I find petting an animal very relaxing and therapeutic. A lot of you may have pets and find them great company. The love an animal gives you is like gold dust and in my opinion, something to be treasured. I often say if humans could have the heart of a dog what a wonderful world it would be.

REST THE MIND AND CALM
YOUR HEART

THE IMPORTANCE OF SOCIALISING

Loneliness is a big problem in society today. It is as damaging to our health as heart disease and other conditions. Loneliness can affect any of us at any time and at any age. It is not only the elderly who get lonely. In modern society people are mixing less and less with their neighbours in housing estates. In winter people tend to stay home more in the dark evenings. By the time you get home from work you may just want to eat and watch TV.

The challenge for us is that social media and phones are getting in the way of communicating with each other face to face. This can lead to loneliness and depression. We need to have social interactions no matter what age we are or whatever limitations we have. Get out if only for a short while. Ring a friend and go for a coffee. Stay off social media if it is upsetting your moods. Choose your connections carefully. I enjoy social media as I have very uplifting connections on there. I unfollow any negative people. My golden rule is "if it lifts you up, keep it, if it doesn't, bye bye." I still limit my time on social media every day.

It is particularly important to know how to connect with people around you so you can fill that need in all of us for a social interaction.

There are a few tips I want to give you today, that will prove helpful in relation to connecting with others:

1. When connecting with others, always find out their name and use it. Some of us don't like to ask more than once but if you didn't get it the first time ask again.

2. Make eye contact. This is important. Don't be looking around you while talking to someone. Stay focussed on the conversation and let everything else pass by. This will make your interaction more pleasant for you and the person you encounter. There is nothing worse than talking to someone and they are not paying attention to what you're saying.

3. Ask their opinion on things, e.g. what is your opinion on… or what do you think about…

4. Touch. When talking to someone or greeting someone, shake their hand or touch their shoulder. A hand sandwich is used the world over and is very effective. It is when you shake hands, and you use the second hand to cover their hand. You also will see the handshake with the elbow touch or shoulder touch. I realise times are changing and shaking hands may not be the done thing anymore but find something that works for you and use it.

5. Smile. A real smile is worth its weight in gold. The power of a smile can lift a person's day. Be warm and approachable when dealing with others. You've all heard the stories of the people who said a pleasant interaction with others saved their lives.

6. Be playful. There is a time and place to be serious, otherwise it is ok to be playful and don't take things too seriously. Have a good belly laugh often as it lifts the soul. I'm not saying be completely airy fairy but enjoy yourself and have a laugh, but not at other's expense.

7. Wisdom needs to be learnt and shared so if it's asked for, share.

8. Listen to others when they speak. Learn from them and enjoy it. It is not easy to do as we often are thinking of what to say next, but with practice you will get used to it. In conversations make sure you're taking in what the other person is saying and letting them finish before you add your opinion. This will help build your relationships and make them stronger.

9. Be kind and calm. Use a smooth, calm voice. This will set a relaxed safe atmosphere.

10. Ask questions. It is always nice to learn about people's lives.

11. Care and understand about what they tell you.
12. Be humble. You don't have to impress.
13. Be yourself. You have nothing to prove. Don't show off.
14. Connect in equal exchange conversation. Don't hog all the air. Let the other person talk as it should be a 50/50 situation. If you are doing all the talking the other person will feel dominated.
15. Praise the other person but don't overdo it. Mean it.
16. Give a compliment where you can.
17. Vulnerability is a lovely quality. Be real and honest about what you are talking about. There is nothing worse than fake people.

YOU ARE THE ARTIST OF YOUR OWN LIFE.
DON'T HAND THE PAINTBRUSH TO ANYONE ELSE.

Communication is divided into 3 areas
7% is what you say and how you speak
38% is the tone of your voice
55% is your body language

Being aware of this will help you a lot. Keep eye contact. Too much can be weird and too little shows disinterest. Don't get easily distracted, stay focused on the conversation. Having good communication skills will help you connect better with people and lead to greater happiness. This is our main goal in life. We are dealing with a lot of challenges so focussing on what brings us joy is a must. I really hope you found something in this book that will help make your life easier as that is what my main objective is. I have been very lucky to have been able to help lots of people and will continue to as long as I have a breath in me. It has brought me so much joy and I am incredibly grateful for that. I believe in sharing what I've learnt if people want it.

Thank you, thank you, thank you to all the people in my life past and present who have listened to me without judgement, helped and guided me without conditions, understood with empathy, and loved me just the way I am through this challenging but wonderful life. I am very lucky to have crossed paths with you all and appreciate your love always.

You are in my heart forever.

REFERENCES

The following references are provided for those readers interested in particular details. A lot of the text in the book is from my own experiences and guidance I have received from individuals I have met over the years. I used notes taken from talks with specialists in the field of M.E./CFS. The following are the references I used.

Completed course in Yale University called Science of Well-Being – by Laurie Santos

Lecture with Dr. Rosamund Vallings MNZM, MB BS Titled Chronic Fatigue Syndrome/ME

Lecture with Dr. Anne MacIntyre on M.E./CFS management. She was a Medical Adviser to the ME Association and the author of M.E./CFS, A Practical Guide.

Documentary. Dr. Anne MacIntyre's Frontline Program about ME/CFS.

Healthline.com

On October 2020, Healthline had a global ranking of 188.

PubMed is a highly respected database from National Institute of Health. It comprises more than 30 million citations for biomedical literature from MEDLINE, and life science journals.

MDPI or Multidisciplinary Digital Publishing Institute is a publisher of author-pays open access scientific journals. It gives information on different areas e.g. Vitamins and what they provide. It has established over 200 broad-scope journals.

Atlasbiomed.com gives details more details regarding all the happy hormones in the Essential Guide to Serotonin and the other happy hormones in your body

The Atlas Biomed Team are makers of microbiome, and DNA test.

Harvard University Medical School. Hormone therapy: The next chapter. Published: March 2011

1912 Casimir Funk did a research publication on vitamins. See hsph.harvard.edu for more.

Conversations with:
Madge O'Callaghan
Dr. Mary Ryan
Dr. Anne MacIntyre
Dr. Rosamund Vallings MNZM, MB BS

Books
- *You Can Heal your Life* - by Louise L. Hay
- *M.e. Chronic Fatigue Syndrome. A Practical Guide* - by Dr.Anne MacIntyre
- *Meditation & Mindfulness*
- *The Secret*- by Rhonda Byrne
- *The Power of Habit* - by Charles Duhigg
- *The Power of Now* – by Eckart Tolle
- *Chronic Fatigue Syndrome M.E.* - by Dr. Rosamund Vallings MNZM, MB BS
- *The Power of Positive Thinking* – by Norman Vincent Peale
- *Emotional Intelligence* – Daniel Coleman
- *The Chimp Paradox the Mind Management* – by Prof Steve Peters
- *Earthing* – by Clint Ober

The Irish M.E. Trust
Carmichael House
North Brunswick Street,
Dublin 7
Lo-call 1890-200-912
Int.tel: 00-353-1-401-3629
Info@imet.ie

Printed in Great Britain
by Amazon

61617049R00113